Advice for Young Doctors

George C Newman, MD-PhD

Chair Emeritus of Neurosensory Sciences,
Einstein Medical Center

Professor of Neurology
Sydney Kimmel Medical College
Thomas Jefferson University

Philadelphia, PA

ISBN: 979-8-9935532-1-4 - Hardcover
ISBN: 979-8-9935532-0-7 - Paperback
eISBN: 979-8-9935532-2-1 - eBook

Library of Congress Control Number: 2025924241

Printed in the United States of America

♾This paper meets the requirements of ANSI/NISO Z39.48-1992 (Permanence of Paper)

1 1 2 5 2 5

To Sally
Who gives meaning to my life
and
Whose Love was big enough to make room for
Neurology

To Matthew and Beth
Who bring joy to my life
and
Who humored my obsession with Neurology

To My Parents
Who gave me the opportunity

To My Teachers, Students, Residents and Patients
Who taught me what I hope to share with you

Acknowledgments

I would like to thank the following people who have read sections of the original manuscript and were kind enough to identify portions of text which were unclear. They have been influential colleagues during my career and most are either a family member or a close friend. The discussions that followed their critiques always lead to improvements in the manuscript and I cannot thank them enough.

In no particular order:
Saman Zafar, MD
Aparna M Prabhu, MD
Tom P Sutula, MD, PhD
Alida M Evans, MD
Heather Newman, MD
Janet O'Sullivan, PhD
Thelma Newman (my 98 year old mother)
Patricia "Trish" Hushen, RN, MSN, SCRN
Brady H Cole, MA, MPH
Margaret V Cole, MSW
Maria V Diaz Rojas, MD
Rabia B Choudry, MD
Henry C Allen, MD, FAAFP
Myriam Poindujour, CNS, RN
Kathleen A Touby BS, RN, MRC, JD
Michael J Glantz, MD
Narges Rahimi, MD
Christine Whelley, RN, NP
Sridhara Yaddanapudi, MBBS, MD
Pooneh M Ardestani, MD
Ignatius C Hazelwood (MS IV)
Teagan McCarthy (MS IV)

Preface

The purpose of this book is to help guide young doctors toward a career that is satisfying for them and beneficial for their patients and patient families. It is an attempt to share some of the lessons that I have learned over a very full career as a physician. This is nothing like a textbook. The topics are based on my own interests with my own biases but, generally speaking, are the topics that my 44 years of practice and teaching have demonstrated to be the topics that excite students and residents, make them feel like doctors and help them to understand and care for their patients. The topics are not as much about information as they are about the process of practicing medicine.

The focus of the book is squarely on caring for patients. From the beginning, the book emphasizes how to learn to maximize your own personal resources, particularly your abilities to interact with people and your thought processes, including the explicit application of logic. You will learn that a short period of reflection on the information already available from your history and exam is often sufficient to make good patient decisions without further testing. Those same logical processes allow you to recognize when more information is needed as well as how to select the most efficient testing strategy to obtain that information.

From the beginning, it will help a great deal if you can learn how to focus your attention on what you are actually doing at any given moment of your practice. There isn't, or shouldn't be, much rote or "knee jerk" thinking in medicine because patients and their problems are infinitely varied. Situations may seem very similar at times but in all of my tens of thousands of patients, I have never encountered two that were the same. No two people are the same and the interaction of host and disease creates infinite variations. Through practice, you will learn to give careful attention to your interactions with patients (and families) while treating their disease processes.

The first "rule" of medicine is often said to be *"Primum non nocere,"* first do no harm. But I think a better first rule was taught to me when I was beginning medical school: <u>You should learn something from every patient you see.</u> If you do just that one thing, with time you are virtually certain to become an outstanding physician. Sometimes the lesson is medical, sometimes it is social or humanistic, and sometimes, if you can be open to it, the best lessons are those that teach you about yourself. With this simple but essential rule, you will learn not only about the diagnosis and treatment of patients, but also about their lives, how to avoid being judgmental, and how to reduce your errors and achieve greater career satisfaction with every patient you see.

All of us who practice medicine recall how bewildering it was at the beginning. That is partly because there are so many abstract concepts that must be internalized along with the overwhelming body of information that must be learned. However, over the years I have come to realize that the abstract concepts can be broken down into smaller and more manageable pieces so that, in the end, learning to apply "the big concepts" of medicine is not much different than learning to start an IV. Success comes through breaking down the complex issues into technical skills that can be learned through practice. For example, there is a chapter on the "Goals of Care" discussions that accompany catastrophic injury or end of life care. In that chapter, the process of managing these intense discussions is addressed operationally. This is the clearest example that I know in which seemingly unmanageable and anxiety-provoking complexity can be broken down into a small number of specific skills that allow you to relax while you help a family organize their thoughts and address their emotions as they go through the process of ***<u>not</u>*** making a decision. What? We'll get to that later.

I wanted to be a doctor when I was four years old and wrote an essay on why I wanted to be a "doctor of the brain" when I was 12. I have had the benefit of knowing and learning from outstanding teachers and colleagues during my career, have had the privilege to help train approximately 200 neurology residents and thousands of residents from other disciplines as well as thousands of medical students from SUNY Stony Brook, the University of Wisconsin, Einstein Medical Center and Sidney Kimmel Medical College in Philadelphia. These residents and students have seen fit to honor me over the years with more than two dozen teaching awards which are among my greatest treasures. So, I must have been doing something right. With this book I hope to achieve the same effects that I did in person. Only time will tell if that is possible.

It should surprise no one that Neurology plays a significant role in this book. After all, I am a neurologist and my experience has been as a neurologist. For this reason, the first chapter, on taking a history, is long and detailed. To an experienced neurologist, obtaining a detailed chronology of the present illness is the necessary first step for diagnosis. However, I want to be very clear at the outset that it is NOT my primary goal to focus on future neurologists. Most of the ideas in this book apply to nearly every branch of medicine. As I tell our Jefferson medical students starting their Neurology clerkship at Einstein, "Our job is not to teach you to be a neurologist, our job is to teach you to be a doctor." In so far as this book is a success, all young doctors will find useful lessons in it.

I learned the logic of clinical diagnosis from the timeless book, "The Early Diagnosis Of The Acute Abdomen" by Sir Zachary Cope. The first edition was in 1921 and the book is still available through Amazon in 2025, more than a hundred years later. That should tell you something about the durable wisdom of the book. Regardless of what type of physician you are or plan to be, if you have never read that book, I strongly suggest that you do so. It is one of the most useful and inspiring books that I have ever read. And you will be comfortable diagnosing a patient who presents with an acute abdomen.

The scope of the present book is determined by what has mattered to me and the young doctors that I helped train. The focus is squarely on diagnostic skills, the process of differential diagnosis, therapeutic decision making, interacting with the rest of your team, and helping the patient to understand and respond to their illness.

I enjoy telling stories and, anyway, "case-based discussion" is the current trend. The discussions will follow my bedside or small group teaching styles as closely as can be achieved in a book. My concern is that "the written word is dead" (Plato) but I will do my best to make it lively. Therefore, you can expect lots of anecdotes throughout, lots of simple and useful sayings from a wide variety of thinkers, a few sayings of my own and, hopefully, a comfortable and entertaining read. Being a doctor can be infinitely rewarding. My goal is for this book to help you enjoy a long satisfying career.

I wish I could stand next to you face to face instead. It would be better by far so that we could share our enthusiasm for the incredible experience of being a physician. Lacking that, here is my best attempt. I hope you enjoy it!

Table of Contents

Acknowledgments i
Preface (Please take a couple of minutes to read this first) iii
Table of Contents vii

1. The History 1
2. Examination 45
3. Fictitious Disorders 69
4. The Logic of Differential Diagnosis 78
5. Therapeutic Decisions 110
6. The "Rules" of Radiology 143
7. Working with Other Physicians, Nurses and Staff 148
8. The Doctor-Patient Relationship 164
9. Prognosis (Predicting Outcome) 177
10. Goals of Care Discussions 186
11. Some Principles of Clinical Pharmacology 217
12. Introduction to the ICU 227
13. Brain Death 241
14. Avoiding Being Judgmental 247
15. Making Mistakes 250
16. Surviving as a student (or junior resident) 253
17. Learn to Teach 262
18. Writing Notes 265
19. Medicolegal Issues 273
20. Causation in Medicine 284
21. Psychiatric Patients 288
22. Interpreting the Literature 294

Epilogue 311

Chapter 1. The History

Introduction to Taking a History.

The patient's history is an essential component in every field of medicine. Neurological conditions are somewhat unique because the patient has experienced the problem directly, and can report accurately (with your help) the symptoms that are the key to the diagnosis. However, just because the patient has direct experience of the symptoms does not mean that they can present that information in a manner that is useful for diagnosis. In fact, the opposite is usually the case. Delving into the patient's experience is much like reaching into my mother-in-law's dresser drawer full of old pearl necklaces in which all of the strings have been intertwined and knotted. It is our role, as clinicians, to separate each string of pearls, lay them out neatly and then line them up so that the temporal relationships among the symptom complexes become apparent.

Put another way, obtaining a history is like reading a William Faulkner novel with multiple stories with overlapping time frames that Faulkner has cut up into short snippets and presented without regard to chronology, frequently shifting from one story to another without any warning or indication. This is how most patients with multiple symptoms will present their history if you let them tell the story on their own. And, of course, multiple symptoms is the rule. The art of history taking requires you to help the patient re-organize their history into each of its component stories, not only with each story in its own chronological order but also sorting which story came first, which ones overlap, and which are the most recent.

Fortunately, there are reliable techniques to address this task. There are usually several ways to obtain a history. Some will be suited to one type of patient and others to different patients or situations. This chapter is about these techniques. The discussion has been shaped extensively by my patients as well as by questions and reactions from students and residents.

The importance of history taking can be illustrated by a study done many years ago comparing diagnostic approaches of junior and senior neurologists. That study identified only one single trait that differed between them. It was not knowledge, or the neurologic exam or even localization skills. The only difference was the greater amount of time that more experienced neurologists spent on the chronology of the present illness.

While the neurologic exam yields a phenomenal amount of information, there are only a finite number of combinations of exam findings which can occur, while the history is infinitely variable, yielding a rich portrait of the patient's experiences as well as their reactions to them. Furthermore, it is often the case that there simply are no abnormal neurologic signs or test abnormalities even after a meticulous work-up so that the information from the history is the only useful data available. This is frequently the situation when the symptoms are transient as in TIA, seizures and headaches.

Naturally, taking a history is simply one part of diagnosis and does not occur in isolation. For one thing, parts of the patient's examination are staring you in the face while you're speaking with them. There is an enormous amount of information that is available to you while you take the history, once you learn how to focus your attention. We'll get to that.

In Chapter 4 we will focus on integrating the questions of our history into differential diagnosis and learn to think of our questions as tests of diagnostic hypotheses.

As compassionate physicians, we should approach history taking with a sense of reverence. We ask patients to share the most intimate details of their lives with us and, in most cases, they do so with an openness that can be disarming even for the most experienced clinician. Their openness proceeds from an expectation of trust that we, as physicians, should hold sacred. Their trust goes well beyond the expectation that we will never divulge the information they shared. At a more fundamental level they trust us to respect their privacy and only ask for personal details that are necessary for their care. Furthermore, as we will discuss further, they trust that we will not be judgmental of them or their behaviors.

With all of that said, let's get on to the "How" of getting a history in operational detail. To convey this operational approach, I am going to suggest many specific questions that I use to elicit information as well as lots of examples illustrating typical question and response sequences. The point is not for you to memorize my questions but rather to make them your own. It is true that the wordings of my questions have been modified over the years to produce the desired result efficiently, but trying to memorize them will lead to a very wooden, inanimate conversation. We don't want that! Instead, as you read, reflect on the stories and details in order to create your own approach to obtaining an accurate history from your patients.

The Setting

The ideal setting is a quiet, pleasant office. Some of us prefer to sit across a desk, facing your patient while other physicians prefer to sit with knees at 90 degrees because they feel that face to face is uncomfortable. If the patient is accompanied by a family member, friend or caregiver, it is best to have that person seated behind the patient out of their field of view so that you can engage more directly with the patient.

Especially during your training, you will often encounter the patient lying on a hospital bed or ED stretcher and there may or may not be a seat for you. Most of us prefer to avoid standing above the patient looking down at them and so, at least, will raise the bed to a greater height. I often lean casually over the ED stretcher rail while avoiding "crowding" the patient. In the ED or hospital, there are often family or friends already present when you approach the bedside.

In any event, you need to be aware of your own presence and appearance. As department Chair, I had the responsibility to help young physicians improve their patient satisfaction scores and I had the opportunity to learn why some physicians were consistently rated highly by their patients. The most common reason that patients were fully satisfied, by far, was that the physician "made me feel comfortable."

Many things contribute to that!

First, no matter how busy, tired, stressed or frustrated you are by preceding events of the day, get rid of them before you enter your patient's space! I literally used to meditate for a moment before entering their room to remind myself that they have come to me for help and that it is my professional responsibility to give them my complete attention and my very best effort. Nothing else matters.

Next, remember that you only get one chance to make a first impression. As soon as you enter the room and for the entire time that you are with them, you need to appear compassionate, confident, professional and focused. They need all of that to get comfortable with you and have confidence in your eventual explanations and advice.

My introduction is always simple. "My name is Dr. Newman, I am one of the neurologists for the hospital." Pre-COVID I always shook their hand (it is a valuable part of the exam) but then didn't. Recently, I find that I have begun to do that again. After all, it is likely that during the visit my hands will be in touch with many parts of their body anyway. But it's not a bad idea to let them see you drying your hands after using the sanitizer as you enter their room.

You also must realize that the patient may or may not be comfortable letting people who accompanied them be present to hear all that they need to tell you. There may be information that they are not willing to share with the others but that they want to share with you. Therefore, I nearly always ask the others to "give me a few minutes alone" with the patient. I tell them not to go far since I will definitely want to hear from them as well. All I want to do when they leave is to ask the patient if they are OK having the others present or whether they would be more comfortable without them. Usually they will say that they do want them present but it is not at all rare for them to wave their hand and respond "they can wait outside."

Which brings us back to the office setting. I really liked going into the waiting room and calling the patient's name. I believe that makes me more approachable, somehow more human and open, since I am willing to perform that simple task. I am "at their service." It also provides me with enormous information as I watch them respond. How is their attention, their hearing, their proximal strength as they arise from the waiting room chair, their own level of confidence or stress, their dependence on the others with them, their gait, their vision, etc? Much more about the essential topic of examination "informal observation" to follow.

We might as well discuss your appearance here. Early in our training period, most of us have very little money for fancy clothes. That is one argument for using scrubs or a white coat, which also help identify our role. My mother judged physicians by how clean they looked. Whether in scrubs, a white coat or "civies", your attire should be neat and clean. Now, we are people as well, so it is our "right" to create our own appearance, including how we wear our hair, piercings and tattoos. What type of clothes we choose is our own affair. However, professionalism requires that you are aware of your appearance. Your appearance will be part of how your patients react to you. That's just human nature and unavoidable, so you have to make decisions about your appearance with that in mind and you need to be aware if earlier activities of the day have left you appearing less fresh and clean than you were when the day started.

Your appearance can also be of use to you. Late in my career, I often said to a student or resident, "You may think that my gray beard gives me a great advantage with the patient, and it does. But I was once young and naive and that was a great advantage too." As a medical student, I was not above pleading for the patient's cooperation during my history and exam so that I "wouldn't get in trouble," making my well being their responsibility. After all, it was often the case that I was helping them while they were helping me. We will discuss the role of acting at the bedside to create an effective bedside manner a little later.

In general, it is best to avoid pins, logos, etc., on your clothes that are not related to your medical center or service. In my opinion, it is a serious error to wear any indications of your political preferences, even if a cause seems really important to you. Why? Because the person may stand on the opposite side of that fence and become offended or, worse yet, focused on your political differences. Again, "professionalism" argues that you should avoid such unnecessary distractions. Especially in a hospital setting, the patient rarely gets to choose you, you just showed up by rotation. Avoiding potentially confrontational slogans on your coat is simply being considerate.

Also, wearing aromatic scents (i.e. perfume or cologne) is wrong, not only because the scent may be offensive to some patients, or distracting to others, but also because aromatics risk allergic reactions, from sneezing to airway narrowing. It's best to avoid those risks.

Whether in an office, procedure room or hospital room, and regardless of what you are wearing, you need to be aware of your posture and actions. Right from the start, I let students who accompany me on rounds know that "If I do something in a room, it is for a reason. If I cross my arms, it is for a reason. If I lean on the windowsill or wall, it is for a reason. And if I pull up a chair and sit down, it is <u>definitely</u> for a reason, so you should think about why I did that in the context of the session." Non-verbal communication is essential to efficient and effective patient management.

Let's take a simple example. I have a gray beard, am 5'6" and wear glasses. Assume that I am in the hospital interviewing a 6'2" 240 pound athletic 30 year old man from a lower socioeconomic strata.

He may be a prominent leader out on the street. If I stand over him with my arms crossed during the interview, speaking with an academic vocabulary in a demanding manner, how can we expect that man to trust me and share sensitive information with me? It would be far better for me to pull up a chair and position myself in a relaxed manner so that he and I are at eye level. I don't need to "talk down" in any way to this man, but I do need to lose my academic jargon and I need to make sure that the purposes of my questions are transparent to him. With those simple measures, I have placed the two of us on equal footing and eliminated any appearance of authority in our relationship. As a child of the '60's, I'm not too keen on authority figures anyway and, with this patient, I'm now in a better position to learn what I need to know in order to help him.

Beginning the Interview

Throughout this book we will focus on the role of acting at the bedside with the goal of "being the physician that this patient needs you to be in order to return to wellness or address their problem." But how do you know what type of physician the patient needs you to be when you are just meeting? Put another way, how do you efficiently get to know your patient during a relatively short patient encounter on a very busy day?

Later in the book we will also emphasize the informal examination and that will help a great deal with this problem but, for now, let's focus on how to start the interview. I've already introduced myself, may have shaken hands, am observing every visual detail available to me and need to start. I also may have asked them to pronounce their last name or taken a stab at the pronunciation and ask them if I said it correctly. I listen and watch as they respond. Lot's of information already, including attention, volume of their voice, accents, etc. If you have time and it's appropriate, you can continue informally and ask where they're from. Soon, though, you have to start getting their information.

I nearly always begin by asking "How old are you?" and then "Are you right handed or left handed?" The first question is always OK, the second reflects my neurology practice. Both questions are simple but require momentary self-reflection by the patient so that the information about who they are starts flowing! Did they understand? Do they need time to reflect on either answer? Is English a second language? Is their answer correct? Their accent, their body language, their attention! Do they turn to an accompanying person (eg - a family or professional care giver) for support? Do they look you in the eye? Are they amused by the simplicity? How confident are they as they interact with you? All that, right there. You are well on your way to understanding what kind of doctor they need you to be. And you haven't even started to hear their story. Based on this, you can already modify your approach to getting the anamnesis (their recollection and narration of their personal history).

I sometimes introduce the main topic simply by saying, "So, what brings you in today?" My wife, Sally, doesn't love that and suggested that I include an intent to help, so, most of the time, I expand that simple line to "So, what brings you in today, how can we help?" I have to admit it puts me and my team in a better light. Note that it is open ended and also avoids the common wise-crack patient responses to opening questions such as 'So, what's the problem?'.

The next words out of their mouth, their response to my simple question, are critical to the encounter. Both the information they provide and the manner in which they provide that information set the focus of your session. Both are infinitely variable and you are now engaged in a unique exercise with a unique patient, a unique problem and a unique reaction to that problem. Hopefully, your response will be unique!

It is not at all uncommon for their response to be different than the reason that you were given from the referring doctor, triage nurse or consult request. That is useful information in and of itself and, if so, you need to understand why there is a difference.

As the patient responds, you are going to have to make a decision about how much time you let them talk without interruption. Some patients are so intelligent, organized and well-spoken that you can let them talk for several minutes without interruption and obtain a useful history. But that is very rare. At the opposite extreme, you may decide to stop the patient after they report their chief complaint and help them organize their history with a series of questions. One patient once said to me, "I see, you're controlling the flow of information." I nodded and responded in a friendly and smiling manner, "That's right." Some physicians try to adhere to a "30 second rule" and let the patient speak uninterrupted for at least 30 seconds. You may need to follow a more controlling process for many different reasons. Some patients have a hard time expressing themselves and do better with lots of questions that require only short answers. Immigrants may not be fluent in the *lingua franca*. But there are also patients who go on without end, wandering all over the place and including lots of details that are irrelevant. And you will encounter people who are lonely and who consciously or unconsciously prolong the interview beyond any reasonable time.

Clearly, the uncommon patient who can narrate their present history is easy and very little needs to be said here, you just need to listen carefully, perhaps interjecting a few quick questions to be sure you understand and encourage them to continue. So let's assume that is not the case and proceed to the patients who need a more active series of questions to obtain an accurate and complete history.

When I use this "many questions" approach, I always warn the patient to let me know if they need a break. "I can wear you out with questions!" They laugh. I laugh but respond, "I mean it, you'll see." Nearly always, within 5 minutes, you will see the patient begin to lose focus and fatigue. At that point, I smile and say, "See, I warned you, I can wear people out with questions. Do you need a bit of a break?" They smile, pause and say, "No, I'm good, we can go on." One patient who was a veteran once told me that providing a particular resident with the history "was worse than being grilled by the gestapo." None of us want that. My little routine helps avoid that and lets the patient know you want to be considerate of their feelings.

Let´s get clear about what we are trying to accomplish during the interview. We want to localize their problem anatomically, discover the pathophysiologies (mechanisms of disease) that are involved, identify the disease involved, determine how best to control the disease process, how best to promote tissue repair and how to ameliorate the patient's symptoms and disabilities. That's a lot.

Then what information do you need from the history for all of this? You need to know their symptoms! You need a subjective description, a detailed time course, the relationships among the symptoms, and the consequences that these symptoms have had for them, as well as any prior diagnostic work-ups and treatments.

The patient has experienced the symptoms. They have the information that we need in order to help them. It is our role to help them express these symptoms in a way that is useful for diagnosis. In addition to the problems already discussed, patients often lack the vocabulary to express their symptoms. Not infrequently, they use terms that differ from our own technical language. Sometimes they may use a word that we also use but they use the word for a very different purpose and with a very different meaning.

A common example of a misleading use of a common term is that patients presenting with Bell's Palsy nearly always complain of "numbness" on their face. As clinicians, we know that the facial nerve's only sensory fibers are on the anterior wall of the ear canal so the term is extremely misleading because the combination of facial weakness and numbness suggests to us that there is a problem in the CNS. Fortunately, on questioning whether they mean that they've lost feeling on their face "like a piece of wood when you touch it," the patient immediately and actively rejects sensory loss. That isn't what they meant at all. But we hear that complaint regularly in Bell's Palsy and in other forms of paralysis. I don't know why they say that. I imagine it has to do with the loss of tone in the paralyzed facial muscles, but that is pure speculation on my part. It is important, however, for us to know whether they really mean sensory loss or not so that we are not mislead in the localization and diagnosis.

This example points out that we must be on guard for "false friends," familiar words that lead us to believe that we know what the patient means when, in fact, we do not. The above example suggests an important tool that we employ regularly to help us uncover those "false friends" and to help patients find the right vocabulary. The device is using familiar descriptive analogies ("like a piece of wood"). We will use this device regularly. It also points out why neurology is very sensitive to a young physician′s culture. Analogies differ in different regions of the country and throughout the world. This is one challenge as you move around during training.

It is, by the way, not necessary or even a good idea to correct the patient's "mis-use" of a word. Nor do we need to correct them when they use their own jargon to express a symptom. Once we understand what they mean, in most cases it makes more sense for us to continue to use their terminology rather than have them learn a new vocabulary. They know what they mean, they have been thinking in these terms since the onset of the symptoms and it makes no sense for us to disrupt their comfort just to make sure they express themselves "properly." What the heck, it is their symptom! Let them call it whatever they like as long as we understand what they mean. OK, sometimes it may lead to future misunderstanding or the patient may already have demonstrated that they prefer to be precisely correct in their language. In such cases, a brief education may be in order, "We call that spinning 'vertigo'." but that is the exception not the rule. It is usually better for us to adopt their terminology.

<u>Helpful Tips: Patient Terminology</u>

1. Make sure you define your patient's symptom terminology, using analogies if necessary.
2. Be aware of "false friends," commonly used words that may not

correlate with our usual technical definitions.
3. Use your patient's own terminology once you have clarified their meaning.

The Chronology

Understanding the chronology, the precise time course, of the patient's present illness is critical for accurate diagnosis. While that may seem obvious, it is worth pointing out several corollaries that derive from this priority. First, we must begin at the beginning! Next, it is useful to know the patient's state of health before their present symptoms began. Also, we need to know when each additional symptom appeared. Finally, we must get a sense of how each of the symptoms has evolved to the present time, which symptoms are accelerating, which ones diminishing and which ones are no longer present at all along with when it disappeared. As we do this, not only do we test our hypotheses of localization and pathogenesis, but we also learn about the patient's present disabilities and priorities for therapy. We also need to determine which additional systemic diseases or injuries have occurred during the symptom progression. That's a tall order!

I have found that to establish the timing of the patient's symptoms it is very useful to think in terms of "epochs" of time. An epoch is a period of time, it has a beginning and an end (which may be the present if it is ongoing). Epochs can also be thought of as time periods that are separated by events. The first event that we encounter in the history is the onset of the Chief Complaint. Even the simplest disease course will have multiple epochs, including the time before the initial symptom onset, the period during which the initial symptom evolved, and the period from when the symptoms were clearly established until the present. There are likely to be other epochs as the Chief Complaint evolves other symptoms appear.

When there are multiple symptoms, there are correspondingly more epochs that need to be defined, especially the time until additional symptoms appeared. Furthermore, different symptoms may evolve at different rates. Even a particular symptom may evolve at different rates over time, more rapidly at the beginning or gradually accelerating over time. It is often the case that patients are aware of having had the symptom for a period of time and then have a noticeable change in a symptom. Naturally, that would form the basis of two epochs, from onset to change and change to the present. In general, thinking in epochs is an important device to help you understand chronology and help the patient narrate the chronology accurately to you. How do you make use of this important concept? How do you define the epochs for the patient so they can provide the information that you need as you help them unravel their history?

We need to introduce another very useful concept, the "anchor." An anchor is the "when" that an event occurs and serves as a reference for organizing the history. An anchor can be any moment to which the patient can relate. It may be the day that the Chief Complaint occurred or the minute it occurred or simply the subjective time that the patient first experienced it. You need to be flexible and find a way to define anchors in a manner that is useful to help the patient establish the chronology.

It's worth exploring this further. Assume that the patient reports that the symptoms started at breakfast. Let "breakfast" be the anchor. We might explore it further by asking, "Do you remember what time it was when you were eating breakfast?" If they don't recall, you still might ask if they were watching TV and what was the show? Had the kids already gone to school or spouse to work? If they recall any of those, you can use the best approximate time. If they don't remember any of that, then "breakfast" itself becomes the anchor. How did they feel before breakfast? How long after breakfast did they call 911 or someone for help? How has their symptom evolved since breakfast? Is it getting better or worse? You see how the anchor serves as a useful time marker that helps you ask questions and serves as a guidepost for the patient as you help them define the temporal sequence.

There are many, many types of events that you can use to establish anchors which then serve to define the epochs of a more chronic history. Holidays are the most common, but specific times such as the beginning of a season, or a birthday, anniversary, graduation, a trauma or the time of a first visit to a doctor for the problem all can work perfectly well. You will often use multiple anchors for a single complex history with several different symptoms because you will need to explore several discrete epochs to define the discrete portions of the chronology. As long as the anchors have meaning to the patient, the patient can handle almost any level of complexity.

Let's see how we might use anchors and their related epochs. "So, if I understand correctly, you were doing really well until Christmas, but ever since then . . ." or "It seems as if most of these problems began around the time you lost your job but then really got much worse after you were infected with COVID." Anchors can be especially useful for exploring the period before the patient's symptoms were first recognized.

Q: "Did anyone at the Christmas party notice that he seemed to be slurring his speech, maybe thinking he was drunk?"
A: "You know, you're right! Several people did joke about that."
Q: "OK. And was he behaving like his usual self? Was he also walking like a drunk or did he seemed confused?" "Was he complaining of dizziness around Christmas?"

Christmas becomes a convenient "anchor" for fixing the time for the discussion of symptoms. More anchors are used for later events.

Q: "Was there any change by New Year's Eve?" "Did you guys celebrate Valentine's Day? Was there any noticeable progression of his slurring by Easter?" "By his birthday in June?"

The anchors need to define epochs that are useful for exploring the symptoms. So each symptom onset defines its own epoch.

Q: "Let me make sure I understand. He began slurring his speech at Christmas, but probably was not staggering. But by Valentine's Day, when your kids came to visit, your daughter mentioned that it looked like he was having a problem with his balance. And then he started having headaches around St Patrick's Day and people were joking about how many beers he had drunk. Is that right?"

The anchors have served to define epochs and the epochs paint a clear picture of what sounds like a developing brain tumor, possibly in the posterior fossa.

Another corollary of this is that it is *absolutely essential* that, for nearly every question that you ask, you specify *when*. The instant that you don't, the patient will answer in a time frame that is different from the one you expect. Just because your last several questions were about the period between Christmas and Valentine's Day does NOT mean that your next question will be answered relevant to that time frame if you do not specify that you are still referring to that period. In fact, it usually will not! The patient is as likely, or more likely, to answer about a different time period, usually one much more recent. Needless to say, that will lead to confusion on your part until you finally clarify with the patient when this unexpected turn of events actually occurred.

Q: "Wait, you say he was having double vision? But I thought you just said he wasn't having any visual problems on Valentine's Day."
A: "Well, he started having double vision a little after Easter."
Q: "Oh, I see. My fault. I wasn't clear. I meant between Christmas and Valentine's."
A: "Oh, no. No, he didn't have any double vision at that time."

Your fault, don't blame them. And don't blame me, I warned you. But you can take comfort in the fact that it happens to all of us from time to time.

Using anchors can provide the patient with a vehicle to give you incredibly precise information around their initial symptoms. "So, when you tried to get out of bed the morning after you were rear-ended, how did your back feel? Were you aware of any . ."

You have to be careful to explore the chronology fully even when a patient uses an anchor and tells you that their problem occurred "since" that anchor. I'll tell you a funny true story that illustrates the importance of obtaining a detailed and accurate chronology.

I was in general neurology clinic at Wisconsin when a patient was referred to me by a surgeon because the patient told him that he had numbness in his left arm "since surgery." Obviously, patients can have complications during surgery although they are blessedly rare. Anyway, I began, along with the patient and the surgeon, by assuming that the numbness was related to the surgery. Seems natural, right? But because I like a precise chronology I used a series of anchors defined in relationship to the surgery.

Q: Were you awake or asleep during surgery?
A: I was out.
Q: OK. When you awoke from anesthesia, was your arm already numb?
A: No (innocently).
Q: Well when you left the recovery room was it numb?
A: No.
Q: By the time you woke up the next morning was it numb?
A: No
Q: How long did you stay in the hospital?
A: About 4 days.
Q: And was it numb when you left the hospital?
A: No, everything was fine when I went home.
Q: Hmmm. Help me out here. When exactly did your arm become numb?
A: I guess it was 2 or 3 months after the surgery.

Now, it is literally true that the patient's problem began "since the surgery" but, at this point, I think that the surgeon and anesthesiologist can relax and feel assured that neither of them has caused any complication. And I can go about my usual business of trying to find out what caused the patient's numbness.

Helpful Tips: Defining When with Epochs and Anchors
1. Define epochs of time marked by anchors to facilitate the chronology of the patient's symptoms.
2. Use the anchors to define the epochs that you explore with the patient.
3. Use external events or changes in the patient's symptoms to "anchor" the time frames early in the session and as you progress.
4. Make sure to specify *when* you are talking about with nearly every question you ask. (Buddha says, "Happiness comes from being careful.")

Talking to the Patient
You want to get the history directly from the patient if possible. That may seem obvious but it is amazingly common to have to silence a loving family member at the beginning of the interview in order to enable the patient to speak. Indeed, having the patient's family in the room may cause the patient to omit a critical piece of the history, eg - "I have AIDS." or "I'm addicted to cocaine." Or "I've been seeing doctors for this for several years but my family doesn't know." This problem arises frequently with children and with adults with communication deficits.

My preference is to bring an adult patient into my office alone and then ask them if they want the accompanying family member to join us or not. While most of the time they will want the person to come in, you will be amazed how often the patient replies, "No, it'll be better to let them stay out there." And that doesn't mean they have something they don't want to share, they may just be glad to have the opportunity to discuss their problem without interruption. As you might expect, bringing the patient in alone often produces an awkward moment in the waiting room but it's worth it to get the information you need. When the patient does want them to join, it's a simple matter to walk out and apologize to the family member but also to let them know that you always like to check because sometimes patients prefer to be alone with the doctor. The family member nearly always understands although some are visibly put out. When the patient doesn't want them, then that's the answer. I usually ask the patient at the end of the session if we can bring the family member in to hear the discussion. Sometimes the answer is 'Yes' and sometimes 'No.' Assuming the patient is a competent adult, it is their choice.

Adolescents are unique, legally children but cognitively closer to adults. And, of course, they have their own concerns, possibly including their parents, other family members or close acquaintances. Unfortunately, they may suffer abusive behavior, although that is comparatively rare. As with an adult, the adolescent should be brought into the room alone initially and given the chance to be interviewed in privacy. Most of the time they decline and prefer to have their parents present. If they say that they do prefer privacy, I usually will go back into the waiting room and explain to the parents that I prefer to begin the interview alone, asking their understanding. In that case, when the interview has been completed, except in particular circumstances specified under HIPAA or Child Protective Services, it is virtually imperative to have the parents in for the discussion at the end of the session. I then provide a summary of what I learned for the parents, without violating implied privacy with the adolescent, and proceed to the discussion of assessment and plan.

What about children? It is possible to get a reasonably accurate description of symptoms from a child as young as 4 years old if the parents will let you "relax into" a conversation with the child. Initially, most young children will tend to cling to and need the support of the parent but by the time the parent has provided the chief complaint and past history, most children will be ready to focus on a conversation with you to describe their symptoms. Having lots of toys on your desk or a nearby play table helps to loosen their grip on the parent for most children.

<u>Helpful Tips: Helping Children Relax</u>

1. Most young children need a few minutes "to check you out." They can't do that while you are looking at them. Therefore, after a brief eye contact and "hello" with a big smile, I usually look away to interact with the parent so that the child has 2 or 3 minutes to size me up. Most children respond very positively to that opportunity.
2. Some children are inconsolable in a doctor's office (we can guess why). For those uncommon times, I sometimes find it helpful to perform a brief "mock exam" with them on the exam table, "examining" them (to no particular value or purpose) while they cry, squirm and resist. This is followed by an authoritatively spoken, "There, we're done!" to finish the mockery and you return the child to the mother. It is amazing how often the child relaxes after that and becomes less anxious and more interactive.

When obtaining a history from a young child, it is very important to have the child focus on you without interruption or fear of contradiction, and therefore it is necessary to have the parent be silent during that portion of the session. This is novel for them and not necessarily comfortable. They do not expect you to interview their young child and so they repeatedly interrupt. A gentle hand up, palm toward them, loosely in a policeman's 'Stop' position, and letting them know that you need to interact with the child for a few minutes will usually suffice. Often a second interruption by the parent will occur "to correct" some perceived inaccuracy and a second gentle reinforcement of your need to hear how their child "understands the problem" is sufficient. Rarely, to make the point, I have had to ask parents if they would be more comfortable going out into the waiting room while I speak with their child. That usually makes the point and they sit back in their chair to let the child speak. Interviewing the child directly is usually very rewarding as it nearly always results in information that was previously unknown to the parent and often leaves the parent speechless when they realize how well their little child can express themselves. Certainly by age 5 years, most children are more than ready to be interviewed. Except for vocabulary, a slower pace and the inflections of your voice, there really isn't much difference compared to interviewing an adult.

Helpful Tips: Interviewing Adults with Impaired Communication

These very same comments may apply to adults as well if they have a condition that impairs communication such as aphasia, severe dysarthria, severe psychiatric disturbance, dementia or global developmental delay. It is frequently the case that a family member "overtalks" the patient who is trying to answer. If the family member interrupts frequently with corrections of minor details, that may make it impossible to establish the flow and rapport with the patient that is necessary to obtain an accurate history. Some patients with difficulty communicating may expect the family member to give the history but, unless the patient is significantly impaired, cognitively or for level of consciousness, this is rarely a good idea as the patient nearly always has useful "internal" information to offer that will otherwise not come to light. The same techniques used to help the parent let the child speak are used in this circumstance. If necessary, I explain to the family member, "I know that much of what he's saying is inaccurate, but it helps me to hear how he understands the problem." I continue, "Your information is really important, and I'm going to want to hear everything you have to say. You can correct everything at the end but please let me speak with him first to understand what he is feeling." If there are further interruptions, I simply look up and stare at the interrupter. They get the message.

Then, when the patient is finished, I turn to the family member and ask, "Did you agree with the basics of what he said? What would you want to change or add." Sometimes it isn't much at all, sometimes it changes matters extensively. Admittedly, in some cases, a few minutes with the patient make it clear that their history is useless because of confusion or difficulty communicating. In that case, I just stop, turn to the other person, acknowledge the limitations and tell them that I will take the rest of the history from them. While most family members are very understanding, every once in a while the family member is seriously annoyed and lets you know it at this point. Fortunately, our professional training helps us understand that this is not about egos so we just accept their expressed annoyance. As Buddha says, 'Learn to respond and not to react.'

Helpful Tips: Hearing Directly from the Patient

1. Unless the patient is cognitively impaired or very young, get the history directly from the patient.
2. Bring the adult or adolescent patient into your office alone at first, and ask whether they prefer privacy.
3. There are techniques to help the patient's family member remain quiet while the patient is being interviewed.

A detailed history of a complicated neurologic problem may take half an hour or longer. The questioning can be very demanding and risks mimicking "Gestapo techniques" if you're not careful. The experience really can be exhausting for the patient, especially one who is very anxious or in active pain. Therefore, as mentioned above, after about 5 minutes of questions, it is important to stop and ask if they are OK. Just break the rhythm and let them clear their head. Ask if they need a drink of water, to shift their weight in their chair, or whatever. "Are you OK?" They always smile and tell me they are "OK" but it helps to let them know that I am aware that this can be difficult and also that I am aware of them as a person and not just a medical problem. In longer histories, I often add one more "check in" for good measure after another 5 to 10 minutes.

It's usually a good idea to make little sounds of acknowledgment while the patient speaks to let them know that you have heard them. "Hmmm", "yea" and "OK" all work fine. If they pronounce an unfamiliar medical term hesitantly, I usually let them know that I know that they mean and then say "Oh, yea. We say . . ." and give the correct pronunciation. Finally, always be on the alert to introduce a subtle joke or pleasantry.

Helpful Tips: Helping the Patient Relax

Find a way of providing opportunities to relax during the interview and to let the patient know that you are aware of them as a person, not just a problem you are solving.

The Chief Complaint

Most of the time, the patient will respond to the question "What brought you in, how can we help?" with their Chief Complaint. Not always, but let's assume that they do. The Chief Complaint provides the focus of your patient evaluation and inquiry. It is your opportunity to learn what it is that concerns the patient and what has brought them to your office or hospital. It is also your opportunity to learn how they think about their problem and so is also an important part of the mental status exam.

The greatest change in my exploration of the Chief Complaint over four decades has been an increasing transparency to help the patient understand and follow the process. Typically, the patient has responded with a symptom ("I have numbness in my right hand") or symptom complex ("I have numbness and some weakness in my right hand, especially when I wake up in the AM.") They may have given you some additional information ("Its been getting worse for the last two months.")

Based on the above discussion, we balance the patient's freedom to speak with focused questions. Generally, I keep the patient's initial statement brief and then explore the complaint, or complaints, in a highly structured manner through a (long) series of questions and answers. Others may give more latitude. It is essential, however, to avoid becoming involved either in a long-winded meandering narrative or a series of Yes and No answers. The Chronology of the Present Illness will eventually provide much more detail. For now we just want to understand the patient's primary concerns and the information that they believe is relevant to that concern.

A useful approach that helps to keep this phase brief but also gives the patient a sense that you intend to be complete is to have them generate a list of complaints. After briefly discussing their Chief Complaint, interrupt gently with something like 'OK, so that's going to be our focus.' or 'OK, we'll come right back to that.' followed by ' What other problems will we need to talk about?' At that point, I literally make a list of their complaints, without any details, by asking 'Anything else?' until they say 'No, I think that's it.' The list only takes a minute to create and provides a sense of the big picture right from the start. It also ensures that you are aware of all of the patient's concerns. The items on the list and the patient's priority for them often provide insight into the seriousness of the Chief Complaint and the urgency involved in this patient's medical problems.

We need to know, of course, when the patient first experienced the Chief Complaint. If they do not indicate the onset spontaneously, it is simple to ask "And roughly when did this start?" or "Roughly how long have you had this?" or "Roughly, when did you first notice this?" Using "Roughly" avoids very time-consuming activities like long discussions between the patient and others present, or going into the purse for the calendar, or phone calls to family at home, etc. For now, you only need an estimate. Plenty of detail will emerge during the History of the Present Illness (HPI). Let's not waste precious time or disrupt the flow of information at this point. The primary use of this approximate date of onset is to guide more detailed questions and to set the stage for obtaining the Past Medical History (PMH). Yes, the PMH.

The Past Medical History (PMH)

It may seem counter-intuitive but after the Chief Complaint and before proceeding to the HPI, I prefer to spend some time on the PMH. In particular, I want to know what the health status of the patient was at the time their symptoms started. That is why it is useful to get the estimate of the time of onset first. Since diseases which become manifest after symptom onset are less likely to play a role in the etiology of the present illness, I usually do not obtain a complete PMH at this point. Instead, in most cases, at this early stage of the history I mainly want to know the medical condition of the patient when their first symptoms began. I complete the PMH later.

Obtaining the PMH in this way takes a bit of skill. As usual, it's a matter of asking the right question in the right way. This is how I like to do it.

> "You say that your symptoms started around December of last year. Well, let's make believe that I met you in November, I know that's before it started, but just stay with me for a minute. Let's assume that I met you in November and asked how your health was at that time. What would you have said?"

Let's pause for a moment because there is actually a lot going on here.

In nearly all cases, the initial response of the patient to my question is to protest that the symptoms began in December, not November. I handle this non-verbally as well as with the above statements. You have to learn to use your face, hands and body to communicate. We will refer to this non-verbal device frequently in this book. It saves enormous time and confusion. So, as I begin to say, "Let's make believe that we met in November, . . ." I am raising both hands toward a modified "STOP" position with my wrists at about 45° and positioned a little above my waist. (I never point my palm at the patient's face to indicate "STOP!" like a traffic cop might do). I push both hands downward 3 or 4 inches twice, like a gentle pump. The overall visual effect of my posture and movements conveys something akin to "Hold on a minute" or a gentle "Whoa." It is very effective at getting them to wait and listen before answering, without being rude. I will recommend this technique many times in this book. I will refer to it as *"Hands in modified stop"* so keep an eye out for it. It is a fundamental technique!

In order to let them concentrate with confidence on your question, they first need to be comfortable that you really mean it, that it isn't just a mistake on your part. Why not just say 'a week before they started'? For some people you can, they will get it, but others will have difficulty grasping what you are trying to do and will be 'more secure' with a more remote time frame. In fact, often something as abstract as a month may not be sufficiently concrete and this will work best when you provide a more specific time. In the present example, a better question might use an anchor and ask them how they were at Thanksgiving or Halloween. Get them to focus back on where they were and who they were with, then ask about their health at that time.

The vast majority of answers from patients will be brief and general, such as 'Excellent', or 'Fine' or 'Not so good.' This actually works quite well for our purpose because it initiates a dialogue. Even though <u>our</u> interest at this point is about their health in general, <u>they</u> are still focused on their Chief Complaint, so they will often respond to our question about how their health was by qualifying their response by adding "But I didn't have any of those symptoms at that point." That's OK, we should expect that and we simply acknowledge that we understand but want to know how they were before their symptoms appeared. Their brief general response is useful because it invites further questions on our part. Begin by acknowledging their response, 'Great' to their 'Excellent' or 'I'm sorry' to their 'Not so good.' Then we proceed to explore in detail. This is not the only time we will set up questions of interest with a preliminary question that eases information flow. Two parts: "How was your health" and then "Tell me more."

If their response was "Excellent" I will continue with "Were you being followed by any doctors for medical problems or taking any medication at that time?" You may be surprised when their answer is Yes and they provide a short list of chronic problems that didn't impact their daily life. If their answer was "Not so good" then I continue by asking for a list of their known diagnoses and ongoing treatments to obtain a reasonably complete PMH right then.

Some patients have very complicated past medical histories and it can be really hard to keep things straight. In these patients, it may help to wipe the slate clean, so to speak, by asking the question, "Well, when was the last time you were completely healthy? This virtually always elicits the perplexed question from them, "You mean *completely* healthy?", to which I respond, "Yes, I mean *completely* healthy. I mean running around, can't keep up with you, not a care in the world healthy." In a patient complex enough to require this technique, your question usually elicits a deep sigh and some thought on their part and then, finally, you get to the beginning of their medical problems. That's the place to start. First, confirm that they had <u>never</u> experienced their Chief Complaint by that time. Then, from that point on, bring them forward in time, chronologically, until you have a catalogue of their medical problems up to the Chief Complaint. Many of these issues will be obviously irrelevant to their problem, some will be obviously relevant and in some, it is necessary to keep judgement in abeyance. Obtain a brief summary of the irrelevant ones, explore the relevant ones in more depth and put the uncertain one "in the parking lot" after a brief description for possible later exploration.

History of the Present Illness

We have already obtained a rough estimate of the time of onset of the Chief Complaint. At this point, it is time for us to begin a detailed discussion of the History of the Present Illness (HPI). It makes the most sense to begin at the beginning.

I like to begin by acknowledging that we have taken a bit of a detour in discussing the PMH. "Ok, good. Now let's get back to what brought you in today. I think you said you first noticed these headaches about a month ago. Is that about right?" Assuming the patient agrees, you may be tempted to accept that date. Bad move! You should always confirm whether the patient's symptoms actually began before the time they suggest. In many cases, their estimate will be accurate but as often as not the symptoms had already been present prior to the stated time. Why? Because the symptoms had occurred long ago and there had been a significant hiatus since the last episode or because the earlier symptoms had been much milder than the presenting episode. Both of these are common.

What is the best way to identify these two situations? We will use the same methods that we used with the past medical history but with the important addition of an additional technique that I like to refer to as "implied skepticism."

You begin by exploring the time immediately before their estimated onset. "You say that the headaches began about a month ago. So, if I met you six weeks ago (or at any established anchor), I assume that you would say that you had never had these headaches before." This simple statement may cause them to correct you. "Well, I had them many years before, but . . ." or "Oh, I've been having them for months but they were much milder than the ones this month." Again, this type of patient response is routine, not at all unusual. But you have to ask.

"Implied Skepticism"

Sometimes your simple questioning will not elicit previous remote or milder symptoms even if they were present. Because this also is common, this is one of the situations to use the technique of "implied skepticism." You set it up by repeating the basic question, "You never had these headaches before?" When they reply, "Never", you respond immediately by asking "Never?" The trick here is to use inflection in your voice to imply that you are mildly surprised by their response, you expected otherwise. If they repeat their denial, depending on the patient and your suspicion, it may or may not be worth one more statement of skepticism, "You *never* had headaches like this when you were a child, you *never* had them earlier, even in a milder form?" Again, there is skepticism in your voice, being careful to avoid being rude. At this point, you can expect either a positive response, "Well maybe, . . ." or a definitive "No, never!" The definitive response is definitive. However, if they give a positive response, you have to be careful because you don't want to put words in their mouth. So if they agree reluctantly, "I don't know, maybe." then you need to treat that response skeptically, it's only a "Maybe."

Symptom Progression

Now that we have a best estimate for the time of onset, we need to understand how the symptom has progressed from then to now. There is a huge difference in defining the progression of conditions which are episodic and those which are not. It is essential, therefore, to determine this aspect of their disease as you begin to explore the symptom progression in detail.

Understanding the details of symptom progression right from the onset is crucial to accurate diagnosis for most clinical entities. I often say to students and residents "If you are going to understand their problem, then you are going to have to understand it at the beginning. And if you don't understand the beginning, then you are not going to understand the problem." To the patient I say, "You can see that I like a lot of detail. So let's take our time with this. I want to hear the whole story!" Now you might think that I am ready to just hear their story at this point. Actually, we are just ready to begin asking questions. So, Hands in modified stop. "First of all, did this come on suddenly or gradually." I often snap my fingers synchronously with the word "sudden" and wave my hand loosely with the word "gradually." As already noted, I am a huge fan of using gestures to help the patient know what I mean.

Symptoms with Sudden Onset

Let's assume that the patient reports a sudden onset. "Ok, can you tell me what you were doing when it started? You were doing what when suddenly . . . what?" Or, "What was the very first thing you noted that wasn't right?" By this time the patient is used to me so they will not be surprised when I listen to their answer and then follow up with another question, "So you were in your usual state up until that moment, right? You were *normal* (emphasis) when you went to bed the night before?"

The presence of new symptoms when a patient wakes up poses a unique problem this may help understand time course and etiology and, for stroke, this may drastically affect decisions about thrombolysis. If the symptoms are reported as present "when I woke up" or "in the early morning", then it is necessary to really drill down to an extreme level of temporal detail. "Let me understand. You were normal when you went to bed the night before. Right? When you woke up, did the symptoms awaken you or did you wake up as usual? Even before you turned over or tried to get out of bed, did you have any sense that something was wrong?" If the answer is yes, you can assume that the symptoms occurred before arousal. If the answer is no, then you still don't know and must continue in micro-detail fashion. "When you tried to get out of bed, was there any problem?" Next, "When you walked to the bathroom were you dizzy, unsteady or notice any difficulty using the toilet, washing or brushing your teeth?" Next, assuming the answer is still "No," then "When you went to make breakfast, was there any problems? Did you have to go down steps to the kitchen?" And on and on, you can see what I'm saying. Step by step until the symptom onset is apparent.

Stroke is not the only condition where onset in sleep or after arousal makes a difference. For example, acute vertigo actually poses similar issues related to etiology determined by precise onset. And is especially important for the diagnosis of benign positional vertigo.

Even after all of this is done we still are not finished with the first episode. As incredulous as this may sound, assuming onset did not occur during sleep, it is worth asking "Looking back on this, did you have any warning that this was coming?" This question provides new information far more often than you would expect after the detailed questions that have preceded it. You might choose to ask some specific questions such as will be discussed in more detail below. For example, asking about transient loss of consciousness, was there dizziness, headache or palpitation, etc.

As I write this and put myself in your place, as the reader, I imagine that you are beginning to think that I am out of my mind. You must also think that I have all the time in the world to see my patients. Well I assure you the latter is not true and I hope the former is not true either, although some have suggested otherwise. Nevertheless, despite understandable skepticism, with just a little practice you will be amazed how easy it is to interact with patients in this manner, how little time it actually takes (far less time than filling out unnecessary test request forms), and how much information the method provides. It moves you quickly forward in your differential diagnosis at the same time that it gains you enormous respect from your patients, who often respond "you are the first person who really listened to me."

We have assumed an acute onset to the symptoms thus far, as opposed to chronic progression. But even symptoms with acute onset can differ in their precise time of progression. For example, ischemic stroke symptoms or the headache of subarachnoid hemorrhage are usually instantaneous. "Like someone flipped a switch (indicating a light switch with your hand)?" Or, "Like someone hit you with a baseball bat (indicating a club-like blow)?" The answer will often be affirmative and makes vascular etiology overwhelmingly likely. Often, however, the symptoms progress over a short but measurable period of time and the patient does not accept the switch-like analogy. In that case, a follow up question is needed. "So from the time you first noticed the numbness, until it was absolutely at its worst, how long did that take?" Stroke may progress over a few minutes but usually not a whole lot longer (although symptoms may recur or new symptoms may appear later with vascular disease). A migraine typically progresses over 15 to 20 minutes and an MS attack or Bell's Palsy usually worsens over an hour or more (even though the patient initially, and understandably, reports the onset as "sudden").

Chronic Symptoms with Gradual Onset

Many times the patient's symptoms have been present for days, weeks, months or years. Once again, knowing details of the progression are critical for creating an efficient differential diagnosis. Consider the obvious difference between symptoms that have been present for two years without changing and symptoms which began two years ago and have been progressively worsening. In the first case it is likely that an event occurred (eg - trauma, a stroke, an acute infection, a psychological crisis) whereas in the second case a malignancy, inflammatory disease, chronic infection or degenerative process, including renal or hepatic disease, is much more likely.

The same techniques used for taking a history of an acute illness also work well for more chronic conditions but let's highlight a few differences. In the first place, the more chronic the condition, the more difficult it is for the patient or family to identify change. To help them explain what has been happening, it is extremely helpful to "drop anchors" as explained above. "Remember how he was at Thanksgiving? Was he like this during the end of summer or had anything changed?" Determining the onset can be particularly difficult. Multiple observers can be extremely useful. "At your daughter's wedding two years ago, did he seem perfectly normal?" Follow a "Yes" with implied mild skepticism, "Completely?" Check on whether there has been any change in activities or lifestyle. "Is he still playing the violin the way he used to?" "Does he read as much as before?" "Has there been any change in his sleep pattern?" "Does he have the same energy and interests as he did when he was 70?" Exploring the reason for life events may help. "I understand he retired two years ago. Was he having any trouble at work that lead to retirement or was he just ready to take it easy?" "When did he and his wife divorce?" "Does he still ask about the grandchildren? Did he remember they were playing in a soccer tournament last month?"

When patients deteriorate gradually, there are two distinct patterns that the patient or family may recognize. These two patterns tend to be associated with different mechanisms of disease so they are worth distinguishing. The first pattern is a slow continuous ramp-like decline, the second is a saltatory, or step-wise, pattern. With the right questioning, the patient or family can usually identify which description is more appropriate. Here's a good example of how it helps to use your hands and body. Transparency also helps. "I understand that she has been going downhill for the last 7 months or so. There are actually two ways that people can go downhill. The first way is slow and gradual (indicate with your hand a smooth down-sloping hill), like going down a ramp. The changes are so slow and so small that you can barely tell if there is any change from day to day or even week to week. It's only when you look back that you realize that there has been a change. The second way someone can go downhill is like going down steps. (As you continue, indicate with your hand a stable platform for a short distance and then have your hand and head make a sudden small descent followed by another stable platform. Repeat this pattern several times.) "In this second way, the person is OK for a while but then has a sudden worsening (vertical descent of your hand), then is stable again (show platform) but then has another sudden setback (repeat)." Then you simply ask, "Which pattern seems closer to her case?" The ramp-like pattern is more often associated with degenerative disorders, eg - Alzheimer's Disease, tumors and chronic indolent infections while the stepwise pattern is more typical of diseases with exacerbations such as vascular dementia, MS and certain inflammatory diseases. Either pattern may occur with psychiatric disorders, depending on the disease and the nature of the inciting disturbances.

Recurrent Symptoms

Another common temporal pattern involves recurrent disorders such as headache, epilepsy, cardio-respiratory and GI conditions. How do you discover that the condition is recurrent? By asking of course! For sure, many patients will volunteer that information or even provide it as part of their Chief Complaint. But if not and the episode they describe is short-lived, meaning that the episode had an ending and they had returned to normal, then it is wise to ask specifically, "Was this the only time you felt that way? Has it ever happened before?" If they answer is yes, then you have your answer. If the answer is no, check at least once using implied skepticism.

With a recurrent pattern, I find it best to do a very detailed description of the first episode using the same approach as with an acute onset disorder. Occasionally I might use the most recent episode instead, especially if that was the reason for presentation. All of the detail is important and it is important to establish that the patient really is describing one specific episode, and not including symptoms from other episodes, using anchor techniques as needed. It is particularly important to identify the patient's ongoing activity when the episode started as it may be a trigger that provides an important clue to the diagnosis. After that, before proceeding to a description of other episodes, I find it more helpful to get an overview of the pattern. "How many times, altogether, have you had these symptoms since that first time?" Many patients will give you a specific answer or best estimate straight away but many patients have a hard time providing an answer or respond with a qualitative response, such as "Oh, a lot." or "Not that often." Clearly, it is more useful to have a quantitative answer, even if only an estimate. I often try simply, "Can you give me a rough idea how many times?" If they still cannot, then there are specific techniques that will elicit an answer. For example, you can ask "Well, would you say that they occur every day, or every week or every month or just every now and then?" Alternatively, another consistently successful technique is to give them an estimate that is ridiculously high, "A couple of hundred times?" The usefulness of this unlikely estimate is that the patient will feel sorry for you because of how wrong you are and correct you with a more reasonable estimate. But sometimes, they nod and say, "Could be." This approach is useful any time you want a quantitative estimate and the patient has a hard time providing that. For example, it might help describing how much weight they have lost, but it is best at establishing frequency or duration. "The pain has been there forever." "Would you say, maybe, 20 years?" "Oh no, not that long. OK, maybe a couple of years."

Here I have left out an important parameter, namely that the frequency of events may have changed over time. Some patients will acknowledge that up front and ask, "Do you mean then or now?" I give them credit. "Good point! Let's talk about both." If I'm on my toes, I'll introduce the possible difference. "OK, so you've been having these spells for almost 7 months. Are they more frequent or less frequent now than they were at the beginning." If the story has been complicated or the patient has difficulty providing specifics, I might use a more explicit separation up front. "Can you give me a sense how often the spells were occurring when they began 7 months ago?" "OK, thanks. And how often have they been occurring this last month?"

At some point, either before or after determining the frequency, I want to know if all of the episodes are the same or if there are multiple patterns or if some of the episodes have unique features. "Tell me, please, are all of the spells the same?" If they say yes, I repeat what they have just told me about the first. "So, you're OK and then suddenly, you hear vague voices and smell smoke, then you feel strange and have a hard time focusing and then you pass out. You're out for 5 - 10 minutes and then you're a bit confused but back to yourself in 15 - 20 minutes. They're all about like that?" Assuming they respond "Yes," then without implied skepticism but with implied empathy, "Have any of the spells been different or had any special features?"

Sometimes, the patient will let you know that the episodes are not all the same. In that case, you need to determine the spectrum of symptoms. I would begin by asking if there are "just a few patterns that repeat" or "are all the spells unique?" In either case, the only way that I know to approach the presence of differing patterns is to ask about the spells one after another. "We're gone over what happened the first time, in March, pretty well I think. You said that your second spell was in May. Let's walk through what happened then. Tell me how it was similar or how it was different from the spell in March." And don't forget to include the circumstances under which the spells occurred. If the spells differ in detail, but they all occur at 10AM after taking all of their BP meds at 8AM, you should have a pretty strong suspicion that the patient is experiencing orthostatic hypotension from their BP medications.

One last comment on temporal patterns of disease. There is a sense in which there can be useful information about the symptom in a negative time period that is, before the patient experienced it or even before their birth, and that has to do with family history. In most cases, it is worth asking whether anyone else in the family has experienced similar symptoms. Headaches, epilepsy, cardiovascular risk, cancers, inflammatory disorders and degenerative disorders all can have heritable components. I mention this here because you might see a time line displayed with a negative value (to the left of the patient's birth) in articles for disorders such as migraine. It is a useful way of thinking.

After all that, what do we actually know about the patient's symptoms? We have the time course, and that is critical, but there is a great deal more that we need to know about their symptoms!

OPQRST

I think it would be useful at this point, to introduce you to a superb mnemonic aid which I first encountered in the classic book on by the father and son team, Degowin & Degowin's Diagnostic Examination. This mnemonic aid is especially useful when addressing the symptom of pain but is generally useful. It is also THE way to organize your questioning when you feel lost regarding the patient's symptoms. My grandson, Zach, was taught it when he trained for ski patrol. The original mnemonic is "PQRST". A decade ago, I found it useful to add "O", so, for me, it is now "OPQRST." Basically, you can feel confident that if you describe the OPQRST of a symptom complex, then you are likely to have all of the information that is available for that symptom. Let's also be clear that you probably will not obtain the information in the order of the mnemonic aid letters but it is a great checklist to guide your questions and especially to be sure you have a complete description of the symptom complex.

Many clinicians do not like mnemonic aids. I'm actually not a huge fan of them myself. This is one of the rare exceptions that I find useful, however. Let's take a look at the meaning of the acronym and then we can expand each part.

O - Other Symptoms
P - Palliative and Provocative Factors (What makes it better and what makes it worse?)
Q - Quality
R - Region
S - Severity
T - Temporal Patterns

We've already covered temporal patterns in detail. Although it is the last letter of the mnemonic, we nearly always start with it. Let's move on.

It might seem to make sense to define the Quality next but Quality is incredibly variable and can be very complex so I often turn to Region and Severity before Quality. The patient usually is ready to volunteer useful information about Region, whether an arm or in the belly or part of the head. But their localization is often less specific than you would like so that further exploration is often needed. The easiest way to proceed is to use your own body and fewer words. With one hand, you can indicate specific patterns on the body. For example, specific nerve roots or nerves follow specific dermatomal patterns whereas brain disorders are often less well localized, perhaps distally or proximally, but not in a dermatomal or neural pattern. You can show them specific dermatomes or nerve patterns while you ask "Was it just one side of your arm, on the thumb side or the pinky side?" "Is the numbness only on the palm side or also on the back of your hand?" "Did it start at your toes and come up your legs?" (Continuously indicating where you mean).

The standard bedside approach to Severity is to use a 0 - 10 scale. I define this for them as follows. "On a scale of 0 - 10, how bad was your pain? (Hands in modified stop.) Where 0 means there is no pain at all (I wave my arms like a baseball umpire would indicate "Safe" while saying this) and 10 is so severe that you are about to pass out, and I MEAN PASS OUT." I slow down and use plenty of emphasis on the capitalized phrase (nodding my head pursing my lips and elevating my eyebrows)." Then I let them respond. (Notice how my body is at work for communication nearly continuously.)

In this system, 1 - 3 is mild and tolerable, 4 - 6 indicates that it can´t be ignored. People usually reach for an OTC pain reliever somewhere around 6-7 and are noticeably uncomfortable around 8-9. Sometimes it helps to check this very subjective scale by asking them how bad their pain is "right now" while you can observe them. A placid person, talking on the phone when you met them and reporting "10 out of 10" is probably not a reliable reporter. If they say "7" or more and look it, I acknowledge their discomfort and let them know that we'll give attention to that ASAP or maybe already have ordered something for them. (Don't forget to check for drug allergies.) Another useful question to judge severity is whether the pain or other symptom interrupts their ongoing activities. A pain of 8 or more is likely to cause them to stop or at least alter their behavior.

It is natural to address "P" at this point, what makes it better and what makes it worse. Simply asking them that question is usually all that you need to do to get your answer. For some patients, it helps to make a few suggestions but it really depends on the symptoms. What might make knee pain better is very different from what might make light-headedness or diarrhea better.

It is likely that we already have some sense of the Quality of the symptom from the Chief Complaint but it is often the case that we need to gain better insight into the quality of their symptoms. The two techniques used for this are specific questions and analogies.

*Example of Lumbar Pain for Asking about **Q**uality*

Let's take lumbar pain ("sciatica") from a herniated vertebral disk as an example. First of all, there are two different types of low back pain which correspond to two different locations of disk herniation, dorsal ("central") or toward the vertebral foramina ("lateral").

Central lumbar disk herniation produces an aching sensation in the mid-back, usually of moderate severity although it can be severe. The aching is present almost continuously. It is usually relieved by lying down and worse when standing, walking, jumping (heaven forbid) or sneezing ("OW", that hurts just thinking about it). There are rarely any "radicular symptoms" which we will describe momentarily but it can produce symptoms of a conus medularis syndrome with difficulty urinating or defecating, possibly with numbness in the feet. (Pain meds and pain itself also lead to constipation however.)

Lateral lumbar disk herniation, on the other hand, usually has less aching but the impingement on a nerve root produces numbness in the involved dermatome and may also produce focal weakness. The usual pain associated with a lateral herniation, referred to as "radicular pain" is a sharp, intense stabbing sensation which usually radiates distally along the course of the nerve. The patients often agree with the analogy that it is "like an electric shock shooting down your leg." The details of the course of this sensation are extremely useful for localization and are usually as reliable or more reliable than the exam or imaging for localization. For example, the upper lumbar roots (L2 through L4, and the related femoral nerve complex) produce symptoms on the antero-medial aspect of the thigh and knee but the lumbosacral roots L5 through S2 produce their symptoms down the back of the thigh following the sciatic nerve. The localization can be exquisitely precise. If the electrical sensation runs to the great toe, the involved root is L5. If it goes to the heel but not to the great toe then it is S1, and if it stops at the back of the knee around the popliteal fossa it is S2. Try and top that with an MRI! I LOVE IT!

Continuing with Q then O

Let's venture into the woods regarding Quality. Pain from mesenchymal organs and viscera tends to be very dull or aching and poorly localized. Since this includes the meninges, blood vessels and most other cranial structures (the brain itself has no pain sensors), headaches are usually dull and poorly localized to the front or side or back, and rarely more discretely. Conversely, if the patient points with one finger to a discrete spot on their head, then the source of the pain is likely to be superficial, probably musculo-skeletal. (Unless they point right between their eyes in which case the likely source of pain is in the pituitary fossa.) On the other hand, "sharp" or "knife-like" pains are nearly always superficial. Throbbing pain is usually vascular, most often from migraine but possibly from vascular disease. Pain from hollow visceral organs is often referred to as colicky, that is, there is a dull basal pain which increases with a squeezing quality. Intestinal obstruction and ureteral obstruction from kidney stones behave this way.

Finally we come to "O", or Other, which stands for associated findings. Patients often have associated symptoms that accompany the Chief Complaint. It is likely that most of these came up during the history of present illness but that isn't always true. Even when it seems that everything has been discussed, one more further search is always worthwhile even if nothing else emerges.

Other associated symptoms are elicited by simple questions such as "What was the next thing you noticed?" This particular question is useful because it continues the chronology of the patient's illness. It helps to know the relationship of subsequent symptoms to the initial symptom, bearing in mind that the initial symptom may not have been the patient's chief complaint.

If there were other symptoms then the question sequence above is repeated. The exact sequence and timing of the second and subsequent symptoms provides extremely valuable information about anatomy and etiology. The simple question, "How long did you have the first symptom before the second symptom appeared?" will usually do the job. The response may be simply, "Oh it was immediate?" In which case I would respond, "At the same time?". To which they will respond either "Yes, at the same time" or "No, it took a few . . ." and give you the appropriate interval. Sometimes, when the symptoms did begin virtually simultaneously, the patient will appeared bewildered before they answer, not just trying to remember but actually confused about how to respond. You can help them out by asking, "Or did they just come at about the same time?"

A closely related and useful question is whether the initial symptom was still present when the second symptom began. It may or may not have been. Again, this can be useful in understanding localization especially in stroke or epilepsy, and occasionally in MS. This can occur, for example, as a result of a migrating thrombus or embolus in stroke or a Jacksonian style march in epilepsy. This information also can provide useful anatomic and pathophysiologic information in any disease process.

After exploring the next symptom, the natural follow up question is "And then what happened?" You explore each symptom and repeat this last question until the patient runs out of new symptoms. But you're still not quite done. After all that, the typical next question is "Was there anything else?" You'll be surprised at how often that elicits still more useful information. That may be hard to believe but you'll see for yourself.

Example of Angina for Using OPQRST

Let's look at angina related to coronary artery disease as an example to analyze a symptom complex with OPQRST.

O - Shortness of breath, nausea, anxiety, dizziness, occasionally numbness in the left arm

P - Made worse by exercise, better by rest

Q - "Pressure", "crushing", "heavy"

R - Substernal, radiating to the left jaw or left shoulder (if it goes to the back then we think about aortic dissection)

S - Variable, from barely noticeable to incapacitating

T - This may have been happening intermittently for quite some time or only recently or even new onset (if it is still present then you better get your act in gear.)

Sensory Symptoms

Sensory disturbances can be even more complex. We've already discussed the term "numb!" You also would want to know "Does it tingle?" "If you rub it gently, is that uncomfortable?" The latter is referred to as a dysesthesia which, according to the gating theory, occurs when one form of somatosensation is lost but other forms in that same region are preserved. This might occur on the soles, for example, in a small fiber neuropathy related to alcohol, diabetes or amyloidosis but can also occur in large fiber neuropathies in which the small fibers are preserved. The common factor of dysesthesias is that one form of sensation is lost while another is preserved.

Sensory disturbances occur in the visual, auditory, olfactory and gustatory systems as well of course. We will deal with visual and auditory symptoms in the chapter on Differential Diagnosis. The most common olfactory symptoms is simply "loss of smell." This occurs frequently after head trauma because shearing forces sever the axons of the olfactory receptors buried in the olfactory epithelium that travel through the cribiform plate to the olfactory bulb. Olfaction may also be lost in chronic smokers and in cocaine abusers or, less commonly from skull base tumors. COVID-19 causes severe anosmia with fair regularity.

Similarly, the most common symptom of the sense of taste is the loss of taste although this is actually quite rare. Recognized causes include cigarettes, upper respiratory tract infections, specific drugs such as antihistamines, allergies, neurodegenerative diseases, aging and zinc deficiency. Complete loss of taste has been a unique feature of COVID-19 infection, occurring in approximately 4 in 10. Dysgeusia, an unpleasant disturbance of taste, can occur in the same conditions as well as with certain medications such as Paxlovid. A particular type of dysgeusia in which food tastes "salty" on one side of the tongue occurs in Bell's palsy when taste fibers within the chorda tympani of CN VII from the anterior tongue are affected but fibers from the posterior tongue of CN IX are intact. Metallic taste can occur with periodontitis. Any condition that alters salivation, including diseases such as local infections of the salivary or parotid gland, Sjögren's Disease or radiation therapy can alter the perception of taste.

Relationship of the History to Differential Diagnosis

This chapter has focused on techniques for obtaining the History of the Present Illness. Because it is already complex and long, the essential discussion of Differential Diagnosis (DDx) has been deferred to a later chapter. In reality however, the two occur simultaneously but I don´t know how to present them simultaneously and I don´t see how you could read or think about them simultaneously. At any rate, it´s my book and that´s how I decided to handle it. We will get to DDx shortly. In that chapter, we will introduce the Review of Systems, not as a list, which is how it is often presented, but rather as an invaluable tool for hypothesis testing in the form of a series of mini review of systems (mini-ROS). The discussion of mini-ROS will also naturally lead us to discuss more common analogies that help our patients describe their symptoms.

What if the Reason for Referral is Not the Patient´s Chief Complaint?

Let's conclude this long chapter by considering the situation in which the patient's stated Chief Complaint is not the reason for which the patient was referred to you. There can be some trivial reasons for this that we can pass over almost without comment. For example, If the patient expresses the same symptom differently; or if they choose to start their story at a different point than the referring provider but eventually arrive at the same point as the most disabling symptoms; or if they acknowledge the presence of the referring reason but consider other related symptoms more disabling. I'm sure you can handle all of these without the need to lengthen this chapter.

I want to focus on a couple of very different situations. First, sometimes when you ask a patient about why they have come and how you can help, they respond "I really don't know." This response is usually associated with one of two very different scenarios. Either they really don't know but their PCP told them they want them to see another doctor, or the other is that the patient is annoyed at being here and is just being uncooperative. The prosody, the rate, rhythm and inflections of their speech usually leave little doubt which is the case. You will recognize the uncertainty in the former and sarcasm in the latter. If the former, that is, that they really don't know, it is often because the PCP has suspicions about a serious condition (cancer, systemic autoimmune process) but isn't sure and/or isn't totally comfortable addressing the condition. They may not want to worry the patient excessively while waiting for your appointment since they aren't sure there is anything to worry about. In the latter case, when the patient is pissed off, usually the referring PCP wants you to help the patient to understand something that the PCP has been unable to convey. For example, in Pennsylvania, you cannot drive for 6 months after a seizure. Period. End of sentence! There are no extenuating circumstances. Or, the referring PCP is recommending an invasive procedure or a complex medical regimen that the patient is reluctant to undertake. Or the patient needs to limit their expectations for long term symptom control. Or something like that.

My own attitude is that, as a consultant, I want to help the referring doctor in any way that they need me to help. We'll return to this later but, for now, I'll simply say that the best way to build a large consulting practice is to be useful to the patient and referring doctor. And if the consultation seems absurdly easy, I follow the advice of Dr. Gary Horowitz, a neurologist and close friend, who taught that "There's only one thing to say when someone sends you a ridiculously easy consult, and that is 'Thank you!'"

One more situation in which the patient's Chief Complaint may not match the referring reason, can occur in the ED. Before I continue, let me be perfectly clear about something. One of my own rules is that I NEVER second guess the providers on the front line. That's a bad idea. Front line providers should never have to worry that people who come after them will be critical. It's way too easy, afterwards, with lots of information and time, to see more clearly what was going on. First line providers, both in the ED and in primary care clinics, are VERY busy and have far too little time and resources for a thorough evaluation. Speaking from the point of view of a consultant, often as the stroke or neurocritical care consultant, I appreciate the opportunity to address a problem early, while it is still treatable or preventable. (I have been the winner of the "Black Cloud Award" for attendings from the Neurology residents three years in a row, since its inception. It's not "bad luck." It is because I encourage early ED consults, before things get out of control.)

But, having said that, there are times when the ED physician will send our service a consult for "facial asymmetry" or "left foot numbness" in a patient who presented with chest pain or symptoms of a URI or constipation. When you ask the patient why they came in, they talk about the chest pain or urinary frequency. Then you say, "Well, your doctor asked us to see you because of facial weakness (or numbness in your left foot)." The large majority of time, the patient will dismiss that complaint. "Ah, I had Bell's Palsy when I was 22." or "I herniated a disk at work several years ago trying to hold up a heavy desk." In such cases, I just confirm that there's nothing new. "You haven't had new problems eating?" You can turn to the person with them, "Do you notice a change in their face?" Or you can ask the patient if they have any new numbness, weakness or pain. If not, a brief exam is all that's needed and a "Thank you" to the referring doctor. However, if the patient does not confirm a prior explanation or is concerned that something has been changing, then its off to work with you. Figure it out.

Chapter 2. Examination

Introduction

You can be excused for expecting that, since I am a neurologist, this chapter on the neurologic exam is going to be long and detailed. But that expectation is not correct. In the first place, there are a lot of good demonstrations on the Internet and that is probably the best way to learn the exam. Secondly, there are already some really well written books on the neurologic exam and there is no reason to add to that excellent list. Instead, the purpose of this chapter is to augment those video demonstrations and texts by pointing out some details that I have learned over the years. In a strange way, this chapter is at once an advanced discussion of the exam and attempt to avoid pitfalls often made by beginners.

Now, if you are reading this book to learn about medicine in general and are not particularly focused on neurology, and honestly I hope that is true of many of you, then you may wish to skip the portion of this chapter devoted to the formal neurologic exam. You will not lose the overall message of the book. However, I think that both future neurologists as well as non-neurologists will find it useful to read through the section on the informal neurologic exam. Furthermore, because the section on the formal exam is intended to be read by someone already familiar with the neurologic exam, if you are not already familiar with it, then I suggest that you view a video on the neurologic exam prior to reading this chapter's section on the formal exam. I will shamelessly promote the Merck Manual video on the exam that was created for Merck by the Einstein Neurology faculty.

https://www.merckmanuals.com/professional/neurologic-disorders/neurologic-examination/introduction-to-the-neurologic-examination

This chapter proceeds with the assumption and expectation that you are, therefore, familiar with the basics of the neurologic exam as well as the general physical exam. Like every other topic in this book, it is not meant to be comprehensive. It is based on my personal experience and is strongly biased by the patients that I have known.

The Informal Neurologic Exam

There is a joke that says that when you get into an elevator with a psychiatrist and say "Good Morning," he or she is thinking "I wonder what he meant by that." That may or may not be true, but I can say for certain that after you shake hands with a neurologist, he or she has already checked the tone and strength of your right hand and arm, as well as your sense of balance, facial expression, eye contact and your sympathetic nervous system. We can't help it. It's hard-wired. That's just one of the reasons that other doctors think that neurologists are weird. I don't even want to begin to tell you what else we will have observed by the time we let go of your hand. I'll just say that if you knew what we knew, you would seem weird too. But never mind that.

The point of this revelation is that the informal neurologic exam, which is done by observation of the patient's ongoing activity when not being formally examined, provides substantial information that is supplementary and complementary to the formal exam that you are taught in medical school. The informal, or observational, exam can confirm or belie findings made on the formal exam. For that reason, and because I assume that you already are familiar with the formal neurologic exam, we will actually begin the chapter with the informal neurologic exam.

Movement disorders are often referred to as "subway diagnoses." There's nothing pejorative in that term. It is used for two reasons. First, the movement disorders are so prevalent that a crowded New York City subway car is likely to have a least one person with a movement disorder. Secondly, as you can guess, visual observation is the key to recognizing movement disorders.

But stroke, MS, dementia, visual impairment, neuropathies, myopathies, brain and spine trauma, psychiatric disorders, inborn errors of metabolism and congenital disorders of development, arthritis, as well as cardiovascular, pulmonary, liver and renal diseases, and many drug side effects, all can provide visible evidence of their presence. So do fictitious disorders. Clearly, it is worth being aware and attuned to these readily available signs that are present during people's every day behaviors and that can provide information that is nearly independent from the signs observed during the formal exam.

Let me ask you a question first. When a patient comes to you for a sore throat and you ask them to "Say, Ah!", do you see that the uvula rises symmetrically in the midline? Obviously you do. But are you aware of that? Maybe or maybe not. But if the patient comes to you for unexplained, painless hoarseness and you ask them to "Say, Ah!", then I hope that you would be aware of how their uvula rises. The patient´s action is the same in either case. It is your focus that differs.

When the patient enters your room, or when you enter their room and they stop what they are doing, do you notice their actions? Their actions are happening in front of you whether you pay attention or not. The point is, that you can learn to pay attention to their actions and, simply put, that becomes your informal neurologic exam. Its there, right in front of you, if you want it.

Now, just because this portion of the exam is informal in the sense described above, doesn't mean that it shouldn't be methodical. You probably could use the same organization as the formal neurologic exam but I prefer to think in terms of the person's readily available activities, including those of our patients. What do humans do that we can observe? Well, they sit, stand, walk, talk, listen, reach for and use objects with their hands. We can also usually infer their understanding of our speech as well as how they interpret their immediate environment. Along with that we can see their mood and attitude toward our presence, assuming they are aware of us.

Consider how you might use a simple structure to analyze a patient with a possible movement disorder. 1) *What is their posture?* What can you observe from their spontaneous movements? Whether sitting or standing, are they symmetric? Is there excess flexion of their trunk and limbs as in Parkinson's Disease? Is there symmetry of the joint angles of their arms and legs? Is their head comfortably centered in the midline? 2) *How are their voluntary movements?* Does their head move fluidly from side to side with their visual or auditory attention? Are the rest of their movements fluid? If on a subway, how do they handle the continuous movements of the car? Do they have the appropriate amount of spontaneous movement, are they blinking, does their facial expression change periodically, do they fidget with their standing or sitting position, shifting weight from foot to foot if standing or cheek to cheek if sitting? 3) *Are there any involuntary movements,* such as tremor of a limb or limbs, or a tic of the face or upper neck and shoulder? Just that minimum structure focusing on their posture and their spontaneous movements is sufficient to guide your observations.

Also, there are two major ways to observe. Either you observe what is happening on its own or you can perturb the system and observe. Simply observing is just that, watch and see what you can learn. To "perturb the system", you can interact with the person in front of you, which is what we do with our patients.

Let's get concrete. If there is someone in the room with you while you are reading this, look up and observe them. What are they doing? While they are doing it, what can you learn about their balance, vision, motor coordination, sensation, motivation? Then speak with them. Ask them what they are doing and observe their reaction. Assuming they stopped and responded to you, what did you learn about their hearing, mood, attitude toward you, language, phonation as well as what they were actually doing?

If there is no one in the room or house with you, turn on the TV and put on any show you want, live or filmed. What can you learn about the people? The answer should be enormous. Of course, you can't interact with them but there are almost certainly others on the show who do. So what do you learn from their responses to those others?

As you do either of these two activities, you are learning how to perform the informal neurologic exam! The idea is that simple. Like anything else, the more you practice the better you will be. If you do it enough, you will be amazed how it enriches your daily life as well as helping you approach your patients.

Let's add more structure to this "informal exam" by looking again at what people do but in more detail. As we watch them, there are things that we observe directly and other things that we infer, some are intermediate between the two. For example, we see their motor coordination directly but we infer their vision as well as their motivation. While we don't directly see their strength, our observations do provide substantial indirect evidence about their strength, especially if there is any weakness. If they are speaking, we hear their phonation, we may infer their intelligence, mood and motivation. Our knowledge of their language abilities also is somewhere in between direct observation and inference.

The informal exam is semi-quantitative at best. Without "perturbing the system," that is, without engaging in the formal neurologic exam, it is difficult to obtain very quantitative information. So, for the informal exam, I suggest that you evaluate each function, whether directly observed, inferred or in between, as either normal, possibly abnormal or certainly abnormal. If you like, you can divide certainly abnormal into whether the abnormality is producing a disability for the patient or not.

Let me remind you that all of this is occurring "on the fly." It should not add time to your patient assessment. You might be speaking with and listening to the ED physician outside the patient's room in the ED, or hearing a resident's presentation, or getting report from a nurse, or some history from a family member. While doing this, you should be observing the patient as nurses, MA or therapists are interacting with them or as the patient is interacting with someone who accompanies them, or while they are using their cell phone, or watching the TV, or watching you and the ED physician, or just lying on the stretcher not doing anything, possibly not even conscious, or conscious but without any initiative. When I am speaking with someone other than the patient, I purposely place myself where I can observe the patient at the same time and I tell the person with whom I am speaking, "I'm listening to you even though I am looking at the patient." And, if the patient sees me and acknowledges my presence, I immediately respond to them with a smile, a nod and a wave, maybe also with "Hi, I'll be right with you" but then I nod to the person with whom I have been speaking so that the patient understands that I am "busy", occupied with other activities. But I don't stop observing them. The amount of information available by observation in this manner is awesome.

When we see someone sitting or standing still, they are not really still. Nearly everyone moves continuously. I am sitting in a park as I write this. The weather is lovely, thank you. As I look up, I can see about 10 people on or near park benches. While I am watching, I see them scratching themselves, shifting weight, brushing their hair, looking around, manipulating cell phones, stretching various body parts. No one is still. In fact, if a person is actually sitting or standing still, you should ask yourself if there are other Parkinsonian features because the odds are that there are. All of these spontaneous movements provide information about the person's gross and fine motor skills, their truncal balance, hints of their sensation, vision and often hearing, their level of consciousness and attention. Facial symmetry is assessable. Then, if they actually do something purposeful, even more info becomes available. If they speak, a whole new class of behaviors presents themselves for assessment.

If I interact with the person, the information is magnified several fold. I call their name. They look at me (because they heard me). They do not lose their balance when they turn. They show recognition or show facial expressions of inquiry (or other reactions they may have to me) and I observe their facial muscles. I can tell much of their mood and/or personality by the speed with which they respond and the fluidity of their facial expressions. They extend their hand or react when I extend my hand, or not. That provides information about their sociability or fear of COVID-19. It provides more information on their balancing ability and their proximal limb control as well as distal strength and tone if we do shake hands. Their sweaty palm tells me they are nervous (or have been recently exercising (which I can distinguish by the state of their clothes). Their vocabulary provides information about their educational level, although less about their intelligence. Of course, their verbal responses also provide information about language impairments. Their logical reasoning skills in response to my queries does provide information about their intelligence as well as their level of attention (or interest about my queries). No wonder you will often hear other doctors say that being a neurologist is like being a detective. In truth we share several skills of history taking and observation. We also share logical analysis of that information. Attention and practice!

Anyway, if I actually walk with someone or observe them walking, then I gain more information about their midline balance and motor skills, the symmetry of their shoulders, arms, hips, knees and ankles with regard to musculoskeletal and neurologic function. Specific abnormalities such as circumducting gait, spasticity, pelvic motor weakness, distal neuropathic weakness, arthritis of the hips, severe scoliosis and pain in their lower limbs are all visible. Endurance, breathing, and angina are observable. If we walk long enough, bladder capacity may emerge.

Enough! You get my point. All of this information is right there in front of you for the taking. It only requires that you pay attention to what is there anyway, whether you notice it or not.

Now the question is, why do this?

What is the value of the informal neurologic exam?

There are two central points. First, you may not be able to get the information from the formal exam because the patient cannot or does not cooperate. Secondly, the findings of the informal exam should be congruent with those of the formal exam. If not, there is something going on that you need to know about.

For the first point, lets take the simple example of examining a four year old child. Some four year olds are capable of being examined like adults but others cannot and few children under age four would be comfortable being examined with an adult's exam. In addition, the formal adult exam provides comparatively little information about a young child. MUCH more information is available from watching the child play. Interview/exam rooms for children are filled with toys. Match box cars, blocks, coloring books and crayons, dolls, action figures and lots of books to look at. Scattered all over the room, including on your desk. Let's see what we can learn. Does the child separate from the mother? Which toy does the child look at first?. How long does the child spend with it? Is the child able to bend down and pick up toys or reach upward for toys? Is the child gentle with the toy or harsh with it, coordinated or clumsy? Can the child attend to a more prolonged activity such as drawing? Does the child pick up a book to read? Does the child avoid the things near to me or does the child come over and look at what I'm doing, even interact with me spontaneously? And on and on. I used to judge the severity of hyperkinetic disorders based on how many times the child turned on the water of the sink in the corner.

A similar point can be made about adults who cannot cooperate with the formal neurologic exam. This can occur because of aphasia, global developmental delay, encephalopathy, depression or anger. It is not rare for the patient to be "uncooperative" for the exam. If you are adept at the informal exam, you can still obtain most of what you need to know. This is true even if they are actively refusing to cooperate.

Fictitious disorders in adults are probably the most common reason for significantly different findings between the informal and formal exams. This topic will be addressed in the next chapter.

General Comments About Physical Examination

I hope that each of you wants to make your patients comfortable, to have them trust you and to have them respect you. Towards those ends, it seems intuitively obvious that we should set a standard of respect, politeness and compassion as we interview and examine them. As far as the exam goes, that means respecting their personal space, minimizing pain and discomfort and letting them know what's coming. Less intuitive is that working quickly, without seeming to be rushed, is also in the best interests of your patient as well as yourself, especially if the patient is uncomfortable.

The Formal Neurologic Exam, General Comments

I am not going to discuss the neurologic exam in depth but want to focus instead on some special circumstances, pitfalls and specific recommendations for the neurologic exam. That'll be long enough.

You have to learn how to adjust your neurologic exam to each patient. Some adjustments are obvious and some are not. For example, we will discuss how to adjust the motor power exam depending on your patient's bulk, general health, age and sex. Your mental status exam has to be adjusted for the community as well as the individual. When I was in Virginia and then in Wisconsin, most of my patients were farmers. When I practiced at Stony Brook, most of my patients were University professors or Brookhaven National Labs scientists, or their families. At Einstein, in Philadelphia, we deal with a diverse Urban population of African-Americans, Jews, Koreans, Latinos and recent immigrants from all over the world. Each community has its own intellectual heritage and cultural standards, and it is necessary for you to adjust your exam to the mean educational level, language abilities and interests of each group.

What is the Point of the Formal Neurologic Exam?
It may seem shocking to ask such a question but I think it is worth considering. First and foremost, the purpose of the neurologic exam is to localize the patient's problem to a given structure in the nervous system, including muscle and the special sense organs. Why? Because different structures of the nervous system are prone to different diseases. There are plenty of examples to illustrate this point. If you find cerebellar deficits on exam, then the patient's dizziness cannot be caused by a disease restricted to the inner ear. If there is evidence of peripheral nerve injury, then MS is probably not the cause. Many excellent textbooks are filled with hundreds of other examples. So, the exam is done to localize the process in the nervous system. The localization within the nervous system greatly narrows the etiologic differential diagnosis, especially when combined with the chronology of the present illness. In addition, the presumed localization on your exam may drive you back to the history to obtain more information based on structures that are "neighbors" of the expected localization. And, the localization strongly impacts your choice of diagnostic tests. If there are no peripheral nerve signs, please don't order nerve conduction studies. If your localization is in the spine, please start with studies of the spine. Obvious, right?

A good examination also is essential to following the course of the disease and response to your treatments. Are the signs lessening with your medication, did the tumor surgery improve their exam or, at least, not worsen the pre-existing deficits. Are they recovering from the trauma? And, by focusing on the neighboring structures of the localized structures, you know which symptoms are likely to emerge next if the disease progresses. That is, it guides your follow-up history and exam, making it more sensitive to progression.

Because different disease processes involve different nervous system structures, the two step process of neurologic diagnosis involves localization and pathophysiology. The legendary neurologist and teacher, Dr. Raymond Adams, was famous for admonishing his residents, "First where is it, then what is it!" Neurology simply is not neurology without following this rule.

You should be aware that it is often possible to elicit neurologic signs with a question. Why would you need to do this? Well, for example, let's assume that the deficit was transient or that patient is no longer ambulatory and you are trying to determine which structures are contributing and which would have been among the earliest signs if you had seen them before they lost ambulation. You could determine if the patient would have had a Romberg sign using questions. How? Well, the point of the Romberg test is that the cerebellum and its connections are reasonably intact but that position sense from the legs and feet are impaired so that when you ask them to close their eyes their stance becomes unstable. So, you could ask them, "When you got up at night to pee, did you have to turn the lights on or hold on to the furniture because your balance was worse than in the daytime?" See how it works?

There are other times that a simple question can provide information that is difficult to obtain on the exam. For example, masseter and pterygoid examination can reveal gross weakness but not mild weakness whereas asking about malocclusion is extremely sensitive to even subtle imbalance of the masseters or pterygoids. You can simply ask the patient "Do your teeth fit together ok when you chew?" Now this is a strange question, for sure, so you also show them what you mean by showing your teeth and slightly opening and closing your jaw, in a gentle "chomp-chomp" motion so you don't have to spend a lot of time explaining.

The Mental Status Exam (MSE)

There are two large sections to the MSE, level of consciousness and content of consciousness. Unfortunately, this duality is often overlooked. Think about it. If you are examining a person who is obviously drunk or stoned, would you conduct a detailed exam involving current events, calculations, abstractions and memory? I hope not. It certainly wouldn't be reliable in the sense of revealing their intellectual capabilities.

We will discuss level of consciousness later in the chapter on ICU but for now let's set some limits. A person is alert when they are actively exploring their environment and anticipating the actions around them. If I examine their right arm and then they hand me their left arm when I put down the right arm, I know that they are alert and that they are a nice person and cooperative. I give them a lot of points for that simple, considerate action. At the other extreme, a comatose patient does not respond to anything. So those are the limits, everything else is in between and we'll put some structure to that when we are in the ICU. Remember that your informal mental status exam has already provided enormous information, usually including their level of consciousness. Are they attentive, agitated, silly, sleeping? We have already discussed the cognitive information that you obtain during taking their history.

Let's assume that the patient is alert or nearly so and proceed to the formal exam of their content of consciousness, which includes their cognitive processes.

The point of the above comments regarding adjusting your cognitive exam to the mean of your community was that by doing so you are able to tell when someone is above or below the norm. You will frequently encounter people of only modest education who are obviously highly intelligent as well as some of similar education who have a degree of intellectual impairment. It is important to know so that you can monitor their disease state but it is also important to adjust the speed and complexity of your explanations when you explain things to them later.

An efficient screening MSE combines multiple cognitive tasks into each test question. If the patient passes the test, then you can proceed but if they fail, then you have to explore the several individual components involved. How fast you go is really important. In general, you want to go as fast as the patient can handle because the speed itself provides a valuable guide to their cognitive abilities and their current level of consciousness. However, you really want to avoid having them make a careless mistake because once they make a mistake, their attention is divided on your next question and rumination on the consequence of their unnecessary error. "Oh no, what will they think of me? I'm so dumb!" If they do that then they are likely to become anxious and inattentive to your next questions, increasing the odds of more errors. You don't want that! How fast should you go? Start with the speed of the history and then consciously accelerate a bit and see if they catch up. (I'm more of an experimentalist than a theorist. So you will often see that I conduct "tests" that guide my future activities rather than trying to predict or, heaven forbid, following a single standard approach that isn't tailored to the individual patient.)

My own MSE that I have used for decades can be seen on the Merck Index video of the Four minute neurologic exam. It is designed to make use of all of the information we gain when taking a patient's history and so tests specific matters which may not be evident from the informal exam as well as providing information that can be used serially to follow the patient's progress.

I test orientation, abstraction, logic, proverbs, right-left orientation, identifying body parts, two step instructions (I don't "command" anyone), calculation, language, sense of humor and memory. Here are a few "technical notes."

For abstraction, I say "Apple, pear and peach. What are they?" I expect an answer of "fruit" of course. I follow that immediately with "Bed, table and chair?" That's it, no instructions! But note the question mark inflection in my voice. There's a lot going on here. First of all, this is a more complex abstraction. Answers can vary quite a bit. The standard response is "furniture" but you'll get a lot of other passable answers, such as "made of wood", "household items" and similar. But a very common answer is "Well, you sleep in the bed, eat at the table and sit on a chair." That's correct but there is no abstraction. You will also hear, "You can sit on them." That's not very good for the table. However, you will also find that quite a few patients just sit and wait for a question. After awhile, they might say, "Well, what?" What's going on here? If I walked up to you on the street and said "Bed, table and chair?" You'd walk away pretty quickly. Then why do most patients respond, "Furniture" when I didn't pose any question? It's because I named three objects in a class (the fruit) and then asked for the class. Then I named three more objects in a more abstract class. They recognized that relationship and assumed I wanted them to name the class. Correct! That's how I simultaneously test logic along with more complex abstraction.

My favorite proverb, by far, is "There's an old saying, 'Don't put all your eggs in one basket.' What's the point of that?" There are many reasons I love this one. First, it is nearly acultural. Even if someone responds "I never heard that one," you can respond "I know but just think about it for a second." I repeat the proverb and ask again. It is also a gradable proverb. I give an A+ to those who respond "Diversify." I'll give an A to those who turn the negative to a positive. You get some beautiful responses that tell you a great deal about the patient. "Keep your options open." A woman with advanced cancer at Fox Chase once responded "There are always many good possibilities." I'll give a B+ to those who correctly interpret the proverb with some abstraction but leave the negative. "Don't rely on one thing." I give a B to "Don't put all your money in one bank." All of these are fine responses. "The eggs might break" is not. If the person can't or won't interpret the proverb, I often try another but, generally speaking, other proverbs are harder. Some proverbs have specific purposes. You can quote from the bible, "Let he who is without sin cast the first stone" to bring some people out of their shell. If you have concern about any psychiatric problem, a good proverb to elicit that tendency is "People who live in glass houses shouldn't throw stones." Finally, just for fun, with a pleasant and advanced thinker, you can use a purposely ambiguous proverb such as "A rolling stone gathers no moss" which depends on your feelings about moss, or the ancient Chinese proverb "In the mind of the novice there are many possibilities, in the mind of the master very few." I'll leave the ambiguities of that one to you.

Right-left orientation, body parts and 2 step instructions are tested simply by asking the patient to "put your right pointing finger on your left ear." Be careful not to let your body or your eyes provide any clues. If they get it right, you've got a lot of good information in a few seconds. If not, you have to figure out what happened. There is an interesting and common response that I call "decomposing two step instructions." The person looks at their finger, confirms it is on their right hand, then almost practices the response of bringing it to their left ear and then fully executes the request. All done correctly, but in multiple steps. This correlates with mild frontal lobe deficits. You will see people place their right index finger on their right ear, or on their nose. Not right. I might repeat with emphasis, "On your left ear." That helps only about half the time. Incorrect responses have myriad causes, often involving the parietal lobe.

Calculation is very community sensitive. At Stony Brook, I asked how much is 20 times 30 and I showed them an "X" with my two index fingers to avoid having them add the two numbers. You'll hear a lot of "500" answers to which I say, "Careful" and they correct the answer. I give them full credit. In Philadelphia, I prefer to ask "If I give you a quarter, a dime and a nickel, how much money would you have?" Many people answer before you finish the question. Many have to take the problem apart, identifying how many cents there are in each coin and adding in two steps. Many never get it right. Unfortunately, there are many people who never learned to calculate, either due to a learning disability or from global difficulty in school.

Language has to be screened. The best screening test for aphasia is naming since nearly all aphasias have difficulty with naming. However, to pass the naming test, the patient must identify not only the object itself, but also a <u>part</u> of the object. This is an essential component and is necessary in order to make the naming test sensitive enough to function as a screening tool. I take advantage of the fact that I wear glasses. I ask them what they are, holding the glasses where the templates meet the rim of the lens and giving them a bit of a shake. You will usually get back "Glasses" but "Spectacles" is still a common response so they get full credit. I then tilt my head back a little, and tap the bottom of the lens. At the same time, I ask "What do you call the part that I look through?" I want to hear "lens." "Bifocals" is also common and totally acceptable. If they respond with "the glass," I return "Yes, but what do you call it?" If I don't get a preferred answer, I'll go on to another object. Possible pairs include Tie and Knot, Belt and Buckle, Cup and Straw or Rim. If they finally get one right, I'm ok but if they never name a part then I proceed to a more complete examination of language.

Humor is a fabulous test of language and logic as well as humor itself. There is no standard "joke" that I use, I always find a way of saying something unexpected and off beat that provides the test. It's also the perfect time to assess the symmetry of their smile! I actively await the right moment or find something to use before I leave the room. From my perspective, the essence of humor is that it is a mis-direction play. You set the person heading in one direction and then suddenly change direction, you pull the rug out from under them. For someone to appreciate the joke, they have to have followed and recalled the initial direction and then recognize the sudden change. Language and logic are both being tested. It's also a way of making yourself a little more human to them and their family.

Finally, for memory, I simply return to the first abstraction. "A minute ago I named three fruit and you told me they were fruit. What were they?" The large majority of patients remember two out of three. If they get all three, I congratulate them and tell them they've "earned extra credit." That may be all the stimulus for testing humor that you need.

I do not hesitate to tell someone that they have performed exceptionally well. Without regard to education, a person who handles speed, earns an A or A+ on the proverb and gets 3/3 objects on memory, is in the top 10% of patients that I see. I let them know that. Why not let them feel good about it? Also, family members who are present usually agree, in which case you get credit for recognizing and acknowledging what they already know.

The Uncooperative Patient

A few words also about the uncooperative patient. More often than not, it is not voluntary. You will encounter intellectual disabilities, encephalopathies, distracting pain, physical injury and incapacitating mood disorders or anxiety, as well as simple "sheer cussedness."

How do you examine them? The informal exam discussed above usually can provide nearly all of the information that you need. However, there is usually additional information obtained from the attempt to examine them. Resistence to motor testing or a threatening gesture provides information about coordination and strength. Please stay alert and be careful! Their refusal to answer a question usually provides enormous information about their language. For people in pain, gentle probing usually reveals at least the site of pain if not the cause and then you can devise a test of motor function that avoids worsening the pain, often an isometric test so the limb and joint are not moved or stressed. It's always a challenge to examine an uncooperative patient but it helps to figure out what you really need to know on exam based on whatever history you have and then design a focused exam around the information that you feel is most important for localization and differential diagnosis. Address the most important exam finding first, you may not get a second chance.

The Four Minute Neurologic Exam

Given the excellent textbooks that already exist and the presence of the Merck Index video on this exam, the rest of this chapter will be limited to very specific "tips" on how to execute the exam most effectively.

Remember that the two most useful purposes of the Four Minute Neurologic Exam are 1) to screen people for neurologic deficits in settings in which no deficits are expected, eg - syncope, headache, seizure, concussion; and 2) to screen the rest of the nervous system in the presence of a suspected very focal peripheral lesion, eg - Bell's

Palsy or radiculopathy.

In order to achieve the 4 minute goal you must use all of the information coming at you, eg - your understanding of their education and mentation during the history and their ability to anticipate what you want them to do; and use your body to "teach" the patient, non-verbally, what you want them to do so as to avoid "false starts" and overcome their inhibitions.

The order of acquisition is designed for efficiency. You will have to sort out these pieces into the 6 fundamental categories at the end:

A. Mental status
B. Cranial nerves
C. Motor
    1. Tone, bulk and strength
D. Sensory
    1. Touch, pin and vibration
E. Reflexes
    1. Deep tendons
    2. Pathologic
F. Cerebellar, gait and station
    1. Station
    2. Romberg
    3. Gait
    4. Tandem

The mental status exam has been addressed above in some detail. I usually postpone the MSE to the end to maximize the patient's relaxation but will move to it immediately if I detect evidence of patient fatigue or if there is suspicion of cognitive impairment when taking their history.

Tip #1. Extraocular movements (EOM).
During visual field testing the patient should be looking at your nose. To transition to EOM, position your penlight in front of your nose (where they are already looking), tell them to "Follow my light" and

move your head out from behind the light. Also, gently place one thumb on their forehead between their eyes, which will prevent them from moving their head.

Tip #2. Facial symmetry.
Resting facial posture is MUCH more sensitive than active facial movements for detecting asymmetry. Put away your flashlight and have them look at your nose. Inspect their palpebral fissures, nasolabial fold and rhizorius muscles for symmetry before moving on to active movements. Inspect the palpebral fissures by observing the amount of white sclera above and below the iris. If one side shows more white, there is asymmetry. Look for a downward slant of the angle of the mouth where the lips meet, to judge the rhizorius.

Tip #3. Trapezius weakness.
Trapezius weakness is most sensitively tested by asking them to shrug their shoulders (demonstrating that for them at the same time). While gross weakness is always obvious, subtle weakness is detected not by testing power but by observing the SPEED with which the their shoulders elevate. Repeat it to be sure if you see a lag. If one shoulder consistently lags behind the other then there is a deficit.

Tip #4. Stick out your tongue.
All of us have an inhibition for sticking out our tongue because our mother's forbade it. BUT, it is OK to stick out your tongue if someone sticks their tongue out at you. So, when you tell them "Stick out your tongue," you stick your tongue out at them. It'll save a lot of time.

Tip #5. Hearing.
I think the Weber and Rinné are almost nonsense. Research shows they are marginally useful when conducted by an ENT physician in a sound proof room. Imagine how reliable they are in the ED! (And your patient will be very unhappy if you follow the Weber and Rinné by using the same tuning fork to test vibration in their feet.)

I test hearing by whispering a number into their ear ("4" in the right ear, "6" in the left) while rubbing my thumb and index finger near the other ear to mask that ear. "1" if a common response to "4", so I accept that as correct.

Tip #6. Grip strength.
You should only put two fingers in their hands when you ask them to squeeze hard. If you put in three and they are strong, your fingers will experience pain.

Tip #7. Arm strength and the importance of leverage.
This is easier to demonstrate than to explain. If you ask a patient to flex their arm to test biceps strength and then pull, you will pull them forward. To avoid this, you must put your other hand on the front of their shoulder on the same side. Similarly, if you tell them to extend their arm to test triceps strength, they will push themselves over backwards. To avoid this, you put your other hand behind their shoulder on the same side.

A fun bedside demonstration involves having a student test my triceps. On first attempt, I begin with my elbow fully flexed. On the second attempt, I begin with my elbow at greater than 90°. On the first attempt I cannot extend my arm. On the second, they cannot prevent me from extending my arm. This illustrates the importance of leverage around a joint. Before testing a muscle, you must decide how to partition the mechanical advantage between yourself and the patient. The goal is to balance the advantage of your relative strengths, so that you have maximum sensitivity to mild patient weakness. If you don't like your first choice, you can always re-assign the advantage and repeat the testing. Every joint has this variable leverage based on the degree of flexion/extension when you initiate the test.

Finally, before I actually engage the muscle I am testing, I give a little tug (toward extension) on the muscle to "wake it up" when testing their flexion or a tap (toward flexion) when testing extension. After the tug or tap, I then engage with full power. Saves time.

Tip #8. Leg strength.

You will often have to examine a patient's strength while they are experiencing local pain, either from spine injury or from limb injury. The general principle is to test their power with an isometric test so the limb is not moving. An especially useful muscle is the extensor hallicus longus (EHL) which is served by the L5 root and peroneal division of the sciatic nerve. With them lying comfortably, ask them to "hitch hike with your big toe" and test the strength by pushing down on the nail bed. It usually takes some effort to overcome the toe and looking for asymmetry increases the sensitivity. Weakness can occur from any lesion from brain, spine, root and sciatic nerve, but you may not be able to test other muscles reliably due to their pain so good strength can be your best screen for long tract injuries.

Tip #9. Achilles reflex.

You must put some tension on the Achilles tendon by gently dorsiflexing the foot passively in order to elicit the reflex.

Tip #10. Babinski reflex.

This is certainly among the most difficult tests of the neurologic exam. The problems are that the patient withdraws from the stimulus and that if you come across the foot too quickly, you can elicit a grasp reflex and hide extension of the great toe. There are some useful alternatives. I like to combine the Chaddock and Oppenheim. The stimuli are a combination of downward pressure on the spine of the tibia above the ankle and stroke the lateral aspect of their foot without moving medially. The response is the same as the Babinski, extension of the great toe and fanning of the small toes. The advantage of this approach is that you can't elicit a grasp by staying laterally and you avoid withdrawal by increasing the pressure on their tibia when they begin to withdraw. They instantaneously learn to stay extended and avoid that noxious stimulus. Also, I always warn them, "I'm sorry, this is really annoying but it has to be done." And do it quickly. Do not warn them that "this will tickle" you will not stand any chance of success if you do.

Tip #11. Quantifying the sensory exam.

I test light touch with a cotton swab, "pinprick" with the broken stick of the swab and vibration with a 128 Hz tuning fork. All of them can be quantified from side to side or proximal to distal very easily. First of all, never ask if the two sides are "the same." The patient will invariably think about it and ask you to do it again. You have to ask if the two sides are "roughly the same." If they note a difference, side to side or proximal to distal, ask which side is less. Then re-apply the stimulus to the normal area and say "If this is worth a dollar," then move to the reduced area and say "then what's this worth?" Nine out of ten times, the patient will provide an answer. You can repeat this with different modalities and different regions. I wish someone would do research on this but have had no takers despite numerous invitations.

Also, don't forget to test double simultaneous stimulation. Simply say and demonstrate simultaneously, "I'm going to touch your right hand (touch it), or your left (touch it), or both (touch both). Just tell me what I touch. Eyes closed (closing your eyes briefly of course and smiling to see if they get the mild joke). Then touch both. If they respond "Both" you're all done. If not, you have more work to do to separate loss of sensation versus neglect. Also, if you know there is partial sensory loss on one side, you can still test for neglect by applying asymmetric stimuli, stronger on the side with sensory loss.

Tip #12. Gait.

Once learned, examination of gait is extraordinarily useful. I ask the patient to walk away from me toward a target (anything will do) at least 15 feet away and then direct them to turn around and return to me. I also clap my hands and ask them to try to hurry "as if you're catching a bus." My observations start at the top and work down, looking for asymmetry: the head and neck, the shoulders, the arm swing, flexion at the elbows, the spine, the pelvis sway, the elevation of the thighs, the flexion of the knees and ankles, how they place their feet.

The "carrying angle" of the elbow is usually about 170°, it is not normal for the elbow to be fully extended to 180°, which indicates some degree of weakness, usually with loss of tone. The pelvis should elevate on the side with the foot raised off the ground. If it falls instead, the patient will walk with a waddle which usually indicates a myopathy. If the entire hip is raised with tilting of the whole body to swing the leg forward to bring the foot off the ground because the knee is not bending, then this is a circumducting gait and correlates with spasticity. Similarly, walking on toes or with a marionette like bounce indicates bilateral spasticity.

As they turn back toward you, any loss of balance will be apparent. I repeat the walk back and forth twice. On the second return trip, I have them stop, take a few steps backwards (indicating with my hand as well as with instructions) and then finish toward me with tandem gait.

And, of course, observe as they arise from the bed or stretcher and return. How natural and fluid are their movements? Do they have to compensate for any deficit?

Tip #13. The Romberg.
This bears repeating at every opportunity due to persistent confusion. The Romberg is NOT a test of cerebellar function, it is a test of proprioception from the feet, ankles and lower extremities. You begin by telling the patient to stand "Like a soldier at attention, heels together" while you demonstrate, gently clicking your heels. If the patient has a midline cerebellar deficit, they will be unsteady and may have to widen their base to remain stable or hold on to something. If they do that, then they have a midline cerebellar deficit (involving the vermis or its connections) and you cannot perform the Romberg. The test would not be valid. However, if they achieve a nice stable position, then ask them to close their eyes (and keep a hand close to them if needed). The Romberg test begins when they close their eyes. You are looking for instability that was not present when their eyes were open. If they had been stable, and then they are not with eyes

closed, then the Romberg sign is positive (or present) and it indicates that there is impaired proprioception from the lower extremities while the cerebellar structures are otherwise intact (because they did well with eyes open). ¿Tiene sentido?

Chapter 3. Fictitious Disorders

There are enough unique features of patients with fictitious disorders that the topic deserves its own chapter. This chapter will also address fictitious coma.

These disorders are relatively common. Patients with fictitious disorders can present to virtually any medical or surgical specialty. They are especially common in the ED, epilepsy clinic and pain clinic, but they also form an important part of the interfaces between neurology, psychiatry and family medicine. As already mentioned, the most common reason for significantly <u>different</u> findings between the informal and formal neurologic exams is a fictitious disorder.

<u>*The Role of Secondary Gain in Fictitious Disorders*</u>
In my simple-minded schema, there are two large categories of fictitious disorders, conscious and unconscious. A conscious fictitious disorder is a form of malingering. An unconscious fictitious disorder is a form of hysteria (to continue Charcot's terminology). (If you prefer, you can also refer to an unconscious fictitious disorder as "a physical or emotional disorder precipitated by severe psychological stress, without other discoverable causes and beyond the immediate control of the patient." That would be much more PC but it is unlikely that the listener will follow what you are saying.)

Personally, I find fictitious disorders of great interest. I believe that the key to understanding fictitious disorders, whether conscious or unconscious, is the patient's secondary gain. For both classes of fictitious disorders, conscious and unconscious, the underlying basis is explained by the secondary gain. Let's explore this important point with two examples, one of my own and one from WWII history.

First, consider an experience of my own, related to malingering. In a period of 3 months, I was called to the ED in the wee hours of the morning for a stroke in a young male patient three times. All three calls were for the same patient and all three visits were the night before he was to appear in court. His formal exam showed unconvincing "give way" weakness. His informal exam, when he was distracted or thinking he was not observed, showed normal motor function. There were no signs of anxiety. By my third middle-of-the-night trip to the ED, I was fed up seeing him sitting there again without any signs of stroke. We notified the police that he would not be admitted and was well enough to attend court the next morning. This was obvious malingering. Secondary gain? Avoiding court. His appearance in court the next day ended his appearances in the ED.

The second example is a classic and commonly cited example of hysteria from WWII. Early in the US involvement in WWII, things were not going well for the Allies. One day, a squadron of six US fighter planes encountered a squadron of six German fighters. Shortly into the battle, five of the American planes had been shot down but the sixth pilot managed to defeat the remaining six German planes. You can imagine that the military seized the opportunity as a way of building morale. So the pilot was returned to the US and hosted all over the country with parades, etc. Eventually, however, he was returned to Europe. When he was climbing into his fighter, his legs abruptly gave way and were paralyzed. How do we explain this? It doesn't take a lot of imagination to understand that he knew what this kind of battle was like, what stress was involved and that he knew that his chances of long-term survival were not great. However, he was the country's hero. He couldn't bring himself to go into battle and he couldn't refuse. Neither option was acceptable. But if his legs were paralyzed, who could expect him to fly a fighter plane? This illustrates dramatically the "double bind" situation in which a person cannot find an acceptable solution and is "rescued" by an unconscious fictitious disability. This type of solution from a double bind is often the unconscious secondary gain of an unconscious fictitious disorder.

I also want to point out that objective evidence has been presented that there is a consistent abnormality in the right parietal lobe of patients with unconscious fictitious hemiplegia that has been observed with PET. Interestingly, the signal is always in the right hemisphere whether the hemiplegia is on the right or left side of the body. So I think that the distinction of "physical" or "not physical" to explain this condition is not very useful. Don't go there. Note that I did not include lack of a "physical cause" as criteria in my description above.

In addressing this situation with the patient, I find it is most useful to let the patient know that we are relieved to find that there is no evidence of injury to their brain or spinal cord, that we don't understand this condition very well, that we do understand that they are not trying to "trick" us, and that most patients with this condition recover relatively quickly. You need to have compassion and set about a plan to help the patient discover and address their secondary gain. A good history is always the place to start. Personally, I always like to ask the help of a colleague from psychiatry as well.

This is a particularly useful approach with non-epileptic seizures, or what used to be called "pseudo seizures." A colleague from Cleveland Clinic has provided evidence to support his hypothesis that non-epileptic seizures are often a form of PTSD. Several of his patients actually appear to be acting out their traumatic event as part of their "ictus." Since learning this from him, I have found numerous examples of my own patients in whom the onset of the non-epileptic seizures is clearly a form of psychological trauma, consistent with his hypothesis.

My approach to non-epileptic seizures for the last 15 years has been based on that concept along with the above information. Consider a patient who has been referred for continuous EEG and video monitoring by a neurologist or epileptologist who suspects non-epileptic seizures. Assume that video monitoring during tapering of drugs appears consistent with that diagnosis, either because there were no seizures or because several attacks occurred and the EEG was unchanged. For simplicity, let's assume that the latter was the case. For this patient, I would recommend continuing one anti-seizure medication since a fairly high percentage of patients with non-epileptic seizures also have epileptic seizures. Then I would sit down with the patient and with their family, if the patient is comfortable with that, and explain the situation as follows.

> This has been a very useful hospital stay. We were able to capture the spells that you had on video and EEG. What we learned is that your spells were not associated with any electrical changes on the EEG so we're pretty sure that these are not epileptic seizures. We call them non-epileptic seizures. We don't fully understand this kind of spell. The situation is usually pretty complicated but they rarely progress to anything more serious and they tend to end on their own. We know that it's not as simple as that you're trying to fool us or that "it's all in your mind" (showing quotes with my hands). They're real enough, its just that we don't fully understand their nature. We know it doesn't make sense to try to stop them by adding more and more seizure medications. That doesn't help and they can make you sick. We do think that you should continue one seizure medicine for a while to be on the safe side and we'll all decide which one together, but only one. In the meantime, we know this whole thing has been very stressful and so I would like you to see one of my colleagues from psychiatry to help you deal with the stress. Of course, we'll see you again in epilepsy clinic, maybe in 4 to 6 weeks, just to see how things are going. Have I been clear in explaining that? Are you OK with what I've said? Do you have any questions or anything you would like to add?

Or something like that. You get the idea.

The Examination of Patients with Fictitious Disorders

Inconsistency is the key to recognizing a fictitious disorder on exam. We have already discussed the importance of discrepancies between the formal and informal neurologic exams. When approaching a patient with a potential fictitious disorder it is useful to observe the patient when they are least aware or to receive a report from another health care team member who has observed both your formal exam as well as their own informal exam. In an ED with curtains separating the beds, it is usually fairly easy to observe the patient informally.

Inconsistency between the formal and informal exams basically means that functions that appear significantly disabled on formal testing are not consistent with the capabilities witnessed when the patient thinks they are not being observed or that are ongoing when you re-enter the room. Typical observations of this type involve texting, walking to the bathroom, talking to others, and using "weak" limbs to reposition themself for comfort or when using the urinal.

Inconsistency is also the key when evaluating the patient′s formal exam as well. There are many possible inconsistencies. For example, the patient shows poor cooperation during history taking. They should certainly want you to find the cause of their problem. Why not be cooperative? Instead they are dismissive of your efforts to obtain a thorough history, consistently responding "I don′t know, I can′t remember" without being disturbed by it. A person with true cognitive deficits is usually pretty upset about being unable to remember something. Similarly, on mental status exam, they don′t make the effort to perform optimally.

Other inconsistencies on exam might include a) inconsistency of motor effort, b) sensory deficits that are inconsistent with known neuroanatomy, c) eyelid fluttering, and d) tearing up during questions (although you also will see patient′s with new deficits tear up at their ability to perform a task, so be careful interpreting that).

There are numerous other signs that each of us develop over the years and are passed on by word of mouth at the bedside. These are not written down for obvious reasons, nor will I divulge my own in writing. Sorry, I hope you understand.

In addition, exams may be inconsistent among consecutive examiners. Compare notes with the other physicians who have seen the patient and see if your findings agree or not.

Finally, a family member or friend accompanying the patient may ask if the problem may be related to anxiety or stress or mood or depression. That doesn't mean it is but it lends weight to the possibility. Also, sometimes you will observe a family member who not only accepts but also supports a diagnosis of stress related symptoms upon hearing your summary and then narrates some recent very stressful life events that the patient has suffered.

Of course, this should not be treated as a "Gotcha" but rather as a more accurate assessment of the situation and probable diagnosis that needs its own unique management.

Remember, the most important factor of diagnosing and treating fictitious disorders is to understand that there is secondary gain, either conscious or unconscious. The second most important thing to remember is that the secondary gain may involve significant psychological stress and that the patient's "fictitious" presentation is really a call for help. You will see patients with many variations on this theme, from recent loss of a child, to exhaustion of a care giver, to physical or mental abuse. These are not trivial disorders to be dismissed lightly, they are doorways into the life of someone who is having trouble coping.

Fictitious Coma

Before concluding, let's apply all of these concepts to the specific condition of fictitious coma. This is not as rare as you might think. Most of these patients will present to the ED but they can also occur in a patient who is already hospitalized.

The term "fictitious coma" is meant to indicate unresponsiveness without underlying injury to the physiologic mechanisms of consciousness including the reticular activating system or cerebral hemispheres diffusely, as will be discussed in the ICU chapter.

One of the most common causes of fictitious coma is a panic disorder due to acute anxiety after the patient experiences an unfamiliar physical symptom such as palpitations or a real or perceived external threat. Patients with Munchausen's syndrome may also present with fictitious coma. To make things more complicated, it is not rare for a patient with fictitious coma to have non-epileptic seizures as well.

In addition to the conscious and unconscious fictitious disorders already discussed, this differential includes physiologic disorders such as narcolepsy and related disorders, and post-ictal states.

The history from an observer often will reveal that a particularly stressful event preceded the onset. There may history of prior anxiety disorders, psychiatric evaluations or hospitalizations. It is useful to ask about prior symptoms of narcolepsy and epilepsy as well.

The examination of coma relies heavily on the eye exam. That is true for fictitious coma as well. If you are not familiar with the eye exam in coma, it may be useful to review that information in Chapter 11 before proceeding here. The pupillary light reaction and consensual light reflex should be present in patients with fictitious coma, of course. In addition, the patient should <u>not</u> have doll's eyes, that is, when you turn their head from side to side for the oculocephalic maneuver, their eyes should follow their head. The eyes will remain fixed in the head, not fixed in space. Patients are not familiar with the oculocephalic reflex so they assume that their "eyes shouldn't work" and so hold their eyes fixed in the orbits as you turn their head. The lack of doll's eyes with normal pupils is the key sign suggesting a fictitious coma.

Another useful sign is to take their limp arms and drop them toward their head. They will virtually always avert their arm enough to avoid hitting themself in the face. In the olden days, when bedpans were metal and ED floors were tile, we used to use the "bedpan test." We would come up behind the patient so they didn't see us and drop the metal bedpan on the tile floor. You cannot imagine how much noise that made. Patients with fictitious coma cannot help reacting to that. A very harsh test which I have never used is cold water calorics. An alert patient will sit up and vomit from the severe vertigo that is induced. That is the definitive test for distinguishing coma but, fortunately, I've never needed to use it.

I really dislike the use of pain in the exam of fictitious coma. First of all, it is MUCH less sensitive than you would imagine. Many patients with fictitious coma do not react to significant pain. I feel awful when I approach a patient with fictitious coma who is bleeding from pinpricks and developing echymoses from noxious stimuli. It also disturbs me, however, because we may be feeding into a psychiatric syndrome similar to Munchausen's syndrome in which the patient is receiving positive reinforcement for a maladaptive behavior. Please don't do that, it isn't useful and it isn't necessary.

Management of fictitious coma is relatively straightforward. As always, begin with ABC. Confirm that vital signs, including respiration and perfusion are all normal. The remainder of my management is based on my own observations that many patients with fictitious disorders had onset as part of a panic attack along with lessons that I learned from Dr. Soo Ik Lee when I was a resident at UVa. By the time the patient hits the ED, they know they are OK but, unintentionally, our medical system traps them into the diagnosis. They can't just sit up and say, "It's all right, I'm OK, I was just frightened. Sorry about the EMS and rescue squad thing." Worse yet, starting IV's, and performing tests, often including a CT scan, prevent them from escaping from the situation. And we do that even though, in many cases, the entire health care team is already rolling their eyes because they can see that the patient is not actually comatose.

When I am comfortable from the history and exam that the coma is fictitious, I simply say out loud, nice and clearly for everyone to hear, especially the patient, "Oh, yeah. I can see what has happened. He's going to be fine. We just need to give him a few minutes to recover." Then I encouragingly rub the patient's arm, speak directly to them and say, "It's OK, you're going to be fine. I'll be back in a few minutes to check on you and watch you recover." And I do. It's important for everyone to avoid snickering and other forms of pejorative speech. Very often although not always, the patient is beginning to "arouse" and interact with the nurse by the time I return. And then I further reinforce their recovery, "Yeah. Perfect! He'll be OK." Often that is all it takes, the patient is ready to leave the ED before all of the tests have returned. Not always though. Certainly there are plenty of times when we have had to admit the patient for "observation." Sometimes the patient is already interacting normally and medically is ready for discharge but is hesitant to leave. I'm fine with admitting them for observation and rarely force a discharge because the patient will find their way back later in the evening. More work for everyone. However, if the patient feels the need to stay and there hasn't been an obvious explanation then, as already discussed, it is important to understand why the patient needed to stay to ensure that they're not avoiding a dangerous threat outside the hospital. You will encounter spouse abuse, "drug deals gone bad" and similar situations under these circumstances.

Chapter 4. The Logic of Differential Diagnosis

Introduction

Diagnosis, identifying the nature of a patient's symptoms, is central to our role as physicians.

Differential diagnosis is the process of exploring a series of possibilities to determine the most likely cause or causes of a patient's symptoms. The "cause" may be evaluated as an anatomic localization, a mechanism of disease, or a specific disease. In most cases, the process is iterative and includes all three.

Note that differential diagnosis explicitly involves likelihood. Osler says, "Medicine is a science of uncertainty and an art of probability." I agree.

The purpose of this chapter is to provide a foundation for the skills of differential diagnosis. The closely-related topic of therapeutic decision making is treated in the next chapter and causation *per se* is addressed in Chapter 20.

There are three themes in this chapter pertinent to diagnosis. The first relates to probability, the second to clinical skills and the third to a series of illustrative examples. Although the three themes are interspersed, earlier sections focus more on logic and probability, the middle is more clinical and the later sections are more case driven.

Testing Hypotheses

Differential diagnosis is, fundamentally, a process of testing hypotheses. In other words, differential diagnosis involves evaluating diagnostic possibilities using a series of if-then statements. For example, if this patient's chest pain is related to coronary artery disease, then it is likely to increase with exertion. All of my experience in practice and as a teacher has confirmed that thinking of differential diagnosis as a series of testable hypotheses is central to understanding, developing and using this critically important skill. Simply put, "Make a hypothesis, test a hypothesis."

This approach emphasizes that differential diagnosis is a VERY active process. Evaluating specific hypotheses helps to guide your questions, the details of your exam and your choices of diagnostic tests. The process begins as soon as you meet the patient but becomes focused by their Chief Complaint.

Because there is no certainty in medicine, it is better to think of hypothesis testing as the process of determining if a diagnosis is more or less likely to be the cause of the patient's symptoms. We are not really "proving" or "disproving" a hypothesis.

Note also that "tests" does NOT refer only to labs, electrophysiology or imaging. A question in the history is a test; seeking a sign on physical exam is a test. Any action that provides new and relevant information about the hypothesis is a test. In fact, the vast majority of your "tests" will be questions and signs The rest are expensive, time consuming and often carry discomfort and risk for the patient.

Example Testing Hypothesis of the Cause of Tremor

A patient presents because of tremor. You hypothesize that the patient's tremor is due to Parkinson's Disease. You test that hypothesis by asking if the patient feels that morning activities of daily living (ADLs) are taking more time and by looking to see if they have masked facies on exam, focusing on the frequency of eye-blinking. See what I mean?

Statistical Concepts of Differential Diagnosis

We speak statistically all of the time in medicine. Just recall prior conversations and notice how often you hear the words "probably," "almost certain to . . .," "possibly," "might be," "unlikely," or "conceivably." It is extraordinarily rare to be completely certain of a diagnosis or to "rule out" a diagnosis completely. We live in a world of likelihood, there is no certainty.

How do we make this art of probability into a science of uncertainty? I explicitly discuss logic and probability all the time when caring for patients whether in the ED, inpatient unit or clinic. So do many other experienced colleagues. It isn't a"teaching exercise," we are thinking out loud. After taking care of patients for decades, that is how we merge the art of probability with the science of uncertainty.

The Universe

I would like to begin by defining "The Universe." Not THE Universe, of course, but a useful concept nonetheless. The patient has presented for some reason; something happened or they wouldn't have come in. Even if it's a fictitious disorder, something has happened. I want to define "The Universe" as the realm of ALL possible reasons why the patient presented. This is a useful start because The Universe has a probability of 100%. Our task is to allocate this 100% among all possibilities. Most diagnoses are irrelevant with probabilities so small that we don't even consider them, but one or more diagnoses will seem probable right from the start.

You may wonder how we can always be sure that The Universe of our differential diagnosis is always 100%, that is, that we haven't missed something. The answer is very simple. We can include a category "Other" which includes everything not in our explicit differential. By acknowledging that it may be something we have not explicitly considered, we ensure that The Universe is 100%, and we ensure humility in our thinking.

How many divisions should there be to The Universe? As many as you want! Whatever is useful. Very often we simply divide The Universe in two. Was this a heart attack or something else? A stroke or something else? But sometimes more divisions are useful. In a patient with unexplained loss of consciousness, a common division would be Syncope, Cardiac, Seizure, TIA or something else. You are free to divide The Universe in whatever manner is useful for the differential diagnosis you are creating for your patient. We will use this concept very frequently so hang onto it.

One way to consider differential diagnosis is that we 1) create The Universe for a patient, 2) estimate the initial probabilities of the potential diagnoses we are considering and then 3) modify those probabilities up or down as we gain more information from the history, physical exam, labs, electrophysiology and imaging. The following discussion provides a pragmatic approach that can be used qualitatively to organize your thinking or quantitatively to produce realistic estimates of the probabilities of your differential diagnoses. The approach is based on applying Bayesian logic to The Universe.

Bayesian Logic in Clinical Medicine

Bayes' Theorem is a marvel of simplicity and power. Basically, Bayes' equation allows us to take an initial estimate of an event (or a diagnosis) and raise or lower the estimate according to whether a test that we perform is positive or negative. In addition, you can string together a series of tests by using the new modified estimate after one test as the starting point of the next test. You can see immediately how incredibly useful that is for differential diagnosis! It intuitively follows our diagnostic process for testing and comparing hypotheses.

As you start asking questions related to the several hypotheses of your differential diagnosis, each time that the patient acknowledges having a symptom or is found to have a sign associated with a particular diagnosis, that diagnosis becomes more likely. When the patient does not have the symptoms and signs of a diagnosis, that particular diagnosis becomes less likely. Now, since The Universe always totals to 100%, when one diagnosis becomes more likely it reduces the likelihood of the other diagnostic possibilities. Similarly, as a diagnosis becomes less likely, the likelihood of all the other diagnostic possibilities increase proportionately. You might say that the less likely diagnosis "gives up" some of its probability to the other diagnoses. We get to use all of the information available about a patient, nothing is considered in isolation. Each feature, present or absent, alters the probability not just for one particular entity but for all other diagnoses as well.

When it is used quantitatively, the final product of this approach is a set of probability distributions for each diagnosis in our differential. But even when the concepts of Bayesian inference are used without any calculations, they provide a powerful and thoughtful approach to clinical diagnosis. Let's explore both approaches.

The conceptually clearest form of Bayes' Theorem for medical diagnosis follows. The equation is stated as Odds rather than as Probability so that it can be expressed as a simple linear equation.

Post-test Odds = Pre-test Odds × Likelihood Ratio
or
$Odds_{Posterior}\,(Disease \mid Test) = Odds_{Prior}\,(Disease) \times LR\underline{+}$

where $Odds_{Posterior}\,(Disease \mid Test)$ represents the odds of having the Disease given the results of the Test; $Odds_{Prior}\,(Disease)$ represents our estimate of the odds that the disease is present before we perform the test; and $LR\underline{+}$ represents the positive or negative Likelihood Ratio. Obviously it will require some discussion to understand and use this clinically, especially about $LR\underline{+}$. But first, does this equation really say that if you estimate the odds of the disease being present and then run a test for which you know the likelihood ratios, that you can calculate the odds that the disease is present in your patient based on the test result with a simple multiplication?

Yes, that is exactly what it says. That's a Wow! Right?

The problem is that, unlike probability, which is intuitive, odds are emphatically not intuitive. An odds of 1 may be the same as 50/50 quantitatively but it certainly doesn't have the same intuitive impact. If I ask you how likely it is that a disease is present in your patient, you will respond 30% or 70% or 90%, or something like that. You will NOT respond, 0.42 or 2.33 or 9 or anything like that. We have very little experience using odds but think, intuitively, in probabilities. Therefore, we want to use Bayes' Theorem in terms of probabilities, not odds, when we use it for diagnosis.

Unfortunately, Bayes' Theorem, expressed as probabilities, becomes non-linear and the calculation is too complicated to do in our head. The solution is either to use Fagan's nomogram or one of the readily available on-line calculators. Eventually, you are likely to rely on a calculator since it is simpler to use and most versions calculate the Posterior probability directly from the sensitivity and specificity of the tests so that you avoid having to calculate the likelihood ratios. However, using Fagan's nomogram and calculating likelihood ratios is extremely valuable as you learn the logic of this diagnostic process because it is visual and allows you to explore how your initial estimate of the disease probability (Prior) and the test's Likelihood Ratios impact your clinical reasoning. I strongly urge you to spend the time necessary to learn this more basic approach before using the calculators in your practice.

In order to use Fagan's nomogram it is necessary to understand the nomogram itself, how to estimate initial probabilities and how to calculate likelihood ratios. So let's do that.

Fagan's Nomogram

It will help for this section to actually have a copy of Fagan's nomogram in front of you. There are many excellent online sources for this. I particularly like this URL: https://jamaevidence.mhmedical.com/data/calculators/LR_nomogram.html .

Fagan's nomogram uses logarithmic scales to compensate for the non-linear nature of probabilities. It usually consists of 3 straight vertical lines. The left line is the Prior, that is, your estimate of the probability that the patient has a certain disease before the specific test is run.

The middle line contains the likelihood ratios. Numbers above 1.0 are used when the test is positive and numbers below 1.0 are used when the test is negative. The right line is the Posterior, that is, the new estimate of the probability that the patient has the disease once we know the LR± and whether the test is positive or negative.

The use of the nomogram is very simple. Using a straight edge, connect your prior estimate on the left line with the positive or negative likelihood ratio on the middle line, and read the results of the Posterior probability for the disease where the straight edge crosses the right vertical line. That's all there is to it.

I suggest that you stop reading here and play with the nomogram for 5 to 10 minutes to see how it works if you are not already familiar with it. Just to confirm that you are using it correctly, here are the results of a few sample calculations for you to test yourself from examples that will be discussed later.

Example #1. Test A has a LR+ of 3.75 and LR- of 0.885.
If your prior estimate is 30%, the posterior estimate is 62% if the test is positive and 28% if the test is negative.
If your prior estimate is 70%, the posterior estimate is 90% if the test is positive and 67% if the test is negative.

Example #2. Test B has a LR+ of 4.5 and LR- of 0.125.
If your prior estimate is 30%, the posterior estimate is 66% if the test is positive and 5% if the test is negative.
If your prior estimate is 70%, the posterior estimate is 91% if the test is positive and 23% if the test is negative.

Example #3. Test C has a LR+ of 12.0 and LR- of 0.04.
If your prior estimate is 30%, the posterior estimate is 84% if the test is positive and 2% if the test is negative.
If your prior estimate is 70%, the posterior estimate is 97% if the test is positive and 9% if the test is negative.

Now that you are familiar with the mechanics of the nomogram, let's discuss how we estimate the Prior probability.

Estimating the Prior Probability of a Disase in our Patients

This is where The Universe becomes explicitly useful. You can divide The Universe in two and estimate the probability of one disease or you can divide The Universe into several sections and estimate the probability of each disease. Naturally, we include Other in either case so the sum of all possibilities in The Universe is 100%.

How do we create those first estimates? The surprising answer is that, with a little practice, you simply learn to do it. It is amazingly intuitive, right from the start. On daily rounds, and many times a day, I poll everyone with whom I am working to estimate Priors; students, nurses, Neurology residents and residents from other services. Everyone. And, of course, I also give my own estimate as well along with other Attendings who are with us. "Ok, the Universe is 100%, something happened. Let's divide The Universe into two parts. Part One, the patient had a seizure. Part Two, it was something else. Together they equal 100%. I want each of you to estimate the probability that this patient had a seizure and then we're all going to say what we think." There is only one rule. "Once you decide, you can't change your estimate after you hear others, otherwise we are not independent." I then go around our group, starting with the most junior and ending with myself, and we say our estimates aloud. What I have learned over decades of doing this is that the MEANS of the three groups (students, residents, attendings) are nearly the same! The difference among the groups is that the variance of the estimates of the group become narrower with experience. But the mean of the students is nearly the same as my estimate, and the same with Neuro or non-Neuro residents. Only the variance changes with group experience. So, there's something about our natural ability, as doctors, that allows us to provide good estimates from the start, as well as to improve quickly with practice.

If you don't like that answer, there is another useful and more rigorous way of estimating the Prior. You can fall back on incidence data. I can illustrate this on rounds easily. Without warning, I can turn to any Neurology resident and ask them the following question. There is a patient in the ED with a stroke. Assuming I don't tell you ANYTHING else, what is the probability that the stroke is hemorrhagic? Without hesitation, they will answer "15-20%." Why? Because that's the percentage of strokes that are hemorrhagic in all large studies and they don't have any other information to modify that statistic so they fall back, naturally and correctly, on the incidence data.

We can make it more complicated but the process is the same. I could tell a Neurology resident that there is a patient in the ED with new onset leg weakness. I don't know anything else but the ED physician thinks it's either due to stroke or multiple sclerosis. I could then ask the resident, without any other information, what is their estimate of the probability that this is MS? They'll have to think for a moment but then they will base their answer on the incidence of stroke in the US (800,000 annually) and incidence of MS in the US (40,000 annually) to estimate that the probability that the patient has MS is only 40/840, or about 5%. So a second approach to providing a Prior, if there is available data and you haven't yet met the patient, is to use the incidences of the conditions in your differential. This is entirely valid.

Anecdotes Illustrating Why It is Useful to Include Other in The Universe

When I was a young child and couldn't find something, my mother would say, "Well if you have looked everywhere that you expect it to be and you still haven't found it, then you're going to have to look somewhere else." That simple truth has guided me many times.

As a first year medical student I was already familiar with the saying "If you hear hoofbeats, don't think of zebras. But then I read a letter in the NEJM that has stayed with me since. In this letter, an internist reported that he and his young son were walking along a city street when they heard running hoofbeats. They turned to see a zebra which had escaped from the zoo. The internist reflected thus.

"Sometimes when you hear hoofbeats it is a zebra. Also, if we had never seen a zebra before, we would not have recognized it." Think about it.

So far so good. We are now familiar with the mechanics of Fagan's nomogram and we have two methods for estimating the Prior probability. The last piece we need in order to apply Bayesian inference is to understand Likelihood Ratios.

Sensitivity, Specificity and Likelihood Ratios

Any time that you read an article about a new diagnostic test, you will always be provided with the sensitivity and specificity of the new test. That is usually the goal of the research that is reported in the paper. For a quantitative test, the paper will usually describe the sensitivity and specificity at some particular cutoff value which is chosen to maximize the area under the receiver operator curve.

Sensitivity and specificity are the primary outcome variables of research related to diagnostic tests but it is hard to know exactly how to apply those two values to a particular patient. For one thing, for some purposes the sensitivity is more important. This is fundamental for screening tests such as syphilis serology, occult blood for colon cancer or mammography for breast cancer. Other times, the specificity is the key as when we are confirming a suspicion of cancer. How do we address this complexity?

One answer is to calculate positive and negative Likelihood Ratios from the measured Sensitivity and Specificity.

We will use abbreviations from the familiar 2 x 2 table.

	Test Positive	**Test Negative**
Disease Present	True Positive (TP)	False Negative (FN)
Disease Absent	False Positive (FP)	True Negative (TN)

We define Sensitivity as the probability of a positive test among those patients who do have the disease,

Sensitivity = TP / (TP+FN) .

We define Specificity as the probability of a negative test among those patients who do not have the disease,

Specificity = TN / (TN+FP) .

The positive likelihood ratio, or LR+, is "the probability that a positive test would be expected in a patient with the disease divided by the probability that a positive test would be expected in a patient without a disease." In other words, LR+ is the ratio of the true positivity rate divided by the false positivity rate, or

LR+ = TP / FP .

The negative likelihood ratio or LR-, is "the probability of testing negative in a patient who has a disease divided by the probability of testing negative in a patient who does not have a disease." That is,

LR- = FN / TN .

We can calculate LR+ from the Sensitivity and Specificity using these definitions,

LR+ = Sensitivity / (1-Specificity) .

Similarly, for LR- ,

LR- = (1- Sensitivity) / Specificity .

Because the ratios involving Sensitivity and Specificity are independent of the prevalence of the disease in the population being tested, so are the likelihood ratios and Bayesian estimates. This is a huge advantage for interpreting tests.

As already noted, it is important to think of questions from the history and exam techniques as tests. Questions and signs also have a specificity and sensitivity, and, therefore, likelihood ratios. Bayes' Theorem and all of the ideas developed in this chapter apply as much to questions and signs as to any other test.

There is one major difference between clinical skills and laboratory tests that illustrates a marvelous distinction between the art of medicine and the science of medicine. When a cutoff value is chosen for a quantitative diagnostic lab test using the area under the receiver operator curve as discussed above, the SCIENCE establishes that there is a necessary trade off between sensitivity and specificity. The more sensitive you make the cutoff value, the lower the specificity and *vice versa*. However, the ART of medicine permits you to simultaneously increase both the sensitivity and the specificity of questions in the history, signs on exam, or the interpretation of visual images from radiology or pathology. I can hear you exclaim "Glory be! Tell me more." I will.

I suspect that when you make rounds with your Attending you eagerly soak up the patient's responses to the attending's questions. And you should. But I also suspect that you don't focus very much on HOW your attending asks the questions. Why is that important? Because experienced clinicians have learned to ask questions in a manner that simultaneously maximizes specificity and sensitivity.

Example Illustrating How Properly Asking Questions Improve Sensitivity and Specificity

We will discuss the concept of focused Review of Systems (mini-ROS) shortly but for now, please take my word for it that the mini-ROS for partial complex seizures involves visual, auditory and olfactory hallucinations, as well as *déjà vu* and fugue states. Here I want to focus on the symptom of auditory hallucinations to illustrate how correct questioning techniques improve both sensitivity and specificity of a question and how getting it wrong does the opposite. It is also an excellent example to make you aware of how sensitive you need to be to the circumstances and concerns of your patients.

Imagine that you are 17 years old and are hearing auditory hallucinations, including the sounds of people talking. Assume that they are related to partial complex seizures that have not yet been diagnosed. However, if you are the teenage patient, based on popular information, what is your own diagnosis? It is that you are developing schizophrenia. So if, I, as the doctor, ask you directly, "Have you been hearing voices?", it is likely that you will say "No, not me." Why? Because you don't want to be diagnosed with schizophrenia, of course, and "be put away" or "have a lobotomy" or whatever doctors do to such people. There goes the sensitivity, the false negative responses are high when asked directly in that manner.

How do we avoid this to regain sensitivity? By being indirect and non-chalant in our questioning. First, wanting to be transparent, I've already told the patient that I am asking questions about seizures and that some seizures are subtle. Also, I NEVER start with auditory hallucinations, Instead I start by asking about visual hallucination. Why? Because visual hallucinations are more commonly associated with "physical" causes such as drugs and the like. So, I might say "Some people with seizures have visual hallucinations. Do you sometimes see things that aren't there or afterwards you decide weren't real?" Then, after exploring that, Yes or No, I move on to auditory hallucinations. "Some people with seizures hear things that aren't there. Could be anything. Could be dogs barking or doors slamming." Then acting nonchalantly and shrugging my shoulders with indifference, I add "Or it could be voices." You can see the person who has been hearing voices relax right in front of you as they begin to describe what they have been hearing. Your sensitivity has been maximized, simply by raising the question in a way that neutralizes their concern about schizophrenia. There are many similar examples in virtually all branches of medicine.

What about specificity? You might ask how we know that the voices are not, in fact, related to schizophrenia. Good question! And there is a surprisingly simple answer.

If you ask someone who is hearing voices because of a psychotic thought disorder whether they know who is speaking, they usually answer that they do. You can ask who and they will tell you. It is usually a relative or close friend, nearly always someone they know or knew. If you ask the patient if they can understand what the person is saying, they will answer that they do. If you ask them what they are saying, they might appear disturbed and be reluctant to tell you. If they do respond, it is often to say something like "It's not very nice." It makes me sad even to write that. How difficult that must be for them.

On the other hand, if you ask someone who is hearing voices because of partial complex seizures, "Do you know who is speaking?" they often look at you in a mildly bewildered manner, as if they don't quite understand the question. When you ask again, they let you know that they do not. When you ask them if they know what the voices are saying, they often laugh and ask you back "Do I know what they are saying?" Amused at their response, you affirm that is what you mean. They laugh again and give you a long, melodic "No." That's because the large majority of patients with seizures who "hear voices" as auditory hallucinations will describe them as a murmuring of a crowd. So, generally speaking, you will have no difficulty distinguishing hallucinations of voices between the two conditions. Ask the right questions and you are rewarded with a high Specificity. Again, there are innumerable examples of how knowing how to ask the question properly improves Specificity. Not only does that get you more accurate information but you also save time by avoiding non-specific information. So, listen carefully as the experienced members of your team interview patients and learn from them. And don't hesitate to ask why they approach the issue as they do if it isn't obvious after the interview. That's how we learn.

Our Bayesian Estimates are Distributions and Not Point Estimates

Let's assume that a Bayesian-oriented attending asks you 'What is the probability of this patient's stroke being cardioembolic?' and you reply, "70%" Do you really mean 70%? Would you accept that it might be 69%? Let's follow this Bayesian conversation on Rounds between a Bayesian-oriented attending (A) and an amused resident (R).

A: You say the risk of cardioembolism is 70%. Could it be 69%?
R: Duh, sure.
A: Could it be 60%?
R: Well, I guess so, but . . .
A: 80%?
R: Maybe, but that seems a bit high.
A: 90%?
R: Not really.
A: 100%?
R: Don't be silly, we are never certain!
A: How about 50%, is that plausible?
R: I don't love it.
A: 40%, is that credible?
R: That doesn't seem consistent with the data.

What is going on here? We see that the resident is not wed to the first response. The attending asked for a point estimate, a single number, and the resident answered the question. But the resident actually would accept a range of answers, some of which are credible and others that are marginal or not credible at all. In reality, the point estimate, 70% in this case, was actually the resident's estimated weighted mean value of a distribution of probabilities. That is virtually always true. In the clinical setting we never believe that there is a single, specific probability that represents the truth of the matter. We just don't have that kind of data for medical diagnosis or medical decision making. We have a range of probabilities in mind and that range is centered around some weighted mean value with a skewed Gaussian-like distribution around that mean. The Estimate actually summarizes a distribution of plausible beliefs. We do this intuitively and we all take for granted what we actually are doing.

In a Bayesian world, what you get is the distribution of probabilities within a credible interval. We then can derive a point estimate in any way that we like, typically we use the distribution mean or median with some skewed Gaussian curve in our mind. There are many ways to do it. Whereas a Frequentist statistician posits that there really is a correct answer, a Bayesian believes that even if there is a correct answer, and there might not be a single "real" answer to a practical question, we cannot know that number. So instead we work with a distribution of possible answers within credible limits based on the data that we have in order to summarize our belief.

Perhaps we should reflect for a moment on why a distribution of beliefs is more appropriate than a point estimate. As alluded to above, the assumptions that we make evolve from information that nearly always includes uncertainties. The history from the patient is more or less reliable. Findings on exam may be equivocal. The diagnostic tests and treatments that we use are never perfect. Osler warned us when he said that medicine is science of uncertainty.

Therefore, behaving like Bayesian statisticians, clinicians work with distributions of beliefs. We use tests to improve our distribution of probabilities, both by improving the estimate of the mean and by improving our confidence in the probability estimates by narrowing the credible limits.

In Bayesian reasoning, the shape of the distribution function is chosen simply for convenience. The distribution is not derived from theory and none is better than any other except insofar as the shape fits the distribution of a particular problem. The normal distribution is often used, especially for typical binomial "Bernoulli" data but there are many mathematical functions that could be used instead, none right or wrong. A distribution function is chosen simply because it fits the data and for no other reason.

When the Data is Unreliable and Distributions are Very Broad

It is important to be conscious of the quality and reliability of the information that you elicit about your patient during the history and physical. Sometimes the patient is confused or has borderline intelligence, or isn't paying attention. Sometimes pain, injuries or other factors limit their ability to cooperate on exam. Witnesses may be vague. You work hard to overcome those challenges and usually can get some useful results, but it would be a mistake to rely upon that information the same way you would when the patient was fully cooperative and the information has been corroborated. I've made this mistake more than once and it almost always leads to the wrong diagnosis. Basically, many factors reduce the Likelihood Ratios for a patient's history and physical signs compared to the average patient. Sometimes you decide that the Likelihood Ratios approach 1.0, meaning you decide that they are virtually useless. When that happens, I do two things. First, I acknowledge the reality of the situation and do not overly rely on the information from the H&P. Secondly, I rely much more than usual on labs, electrophysiology and imaging because they are less prone to error based on cooperation, although not entirely. The patient may not cooperate for blood draws or hold still in the scanner so that even your "objective" information is compromised. Oh, well. It happens. All you can do is be aware of the situation, keep a broad differential and wide distributions for your probability estimates in The Universe.

The take home message is that Bayesian distributions summarize all that we know. That distribution of estimates is all you have to work with. But that's a lot.

Clinical Applications of Bayesian Inference

This way of thinking has wide-ranging implications for differential diagnosis, even if you don't actually calculate probabilities. The rest of this chapter will explore these diverse implications, including with quantitative examples, in order to make you comfortable with the concepts and understand how this approach can sharpen your diagnostic skills. Although most examples pertain to neurologic patients, I will do my best to explain the general implications of each example as we introduce progressively greater complexity.

We will analyze three examples in detail in order to understand the impact of the initial estimate of the Prior and values of the positive and negative Likelihood Ratios (LR+ and LR-) on the Posterior estimates after a test has been run.

Example 1. Moderate Specificity, Poor Sensitivity.
This example explores how the presence or absence of olfactory hallucinations alters the Prior estimate in a patient with unexplained loss of consciousness.

A 19 year old man is being evaluated for transient unprovoked altered consciousness. You learn that right before the spell he had olfactory hallucinations and has been having them for several months. Our focus is on how olfactory hallucinations alter our estimate of the likelihood that the patient has partial complex epilepsy (PCS, also known as focal unaware epilepsy). Olfactory hallucinations have very high specificity for PCS but low sensitivity. I will estimate 96% specificity but only 15% sensitivity for illustrative purposes. From this data we can calculate that LR+ = 3.75 and LR- = 0.885. The LR- is close to 1.0 due to the low sensitivity. We'll vary the *Prior* estimate that the patient had seizures from 10% to 70%. If you wanted to use incidence data for seizures in this setting you might choose a Prior of 10% but if you focus on the recurrence of symptoms you might estimate as high as 70%. We will calculate the Posterior probability using Fagan's nomogram both for the presence and absence of olfactory hallucinations prior to the altered consciousness.

Prior Probability	With Olfactory Hallucinations (LR+)	No Olfactory Hallucinations (LR-)
10%	30%	9%
30%	62%	28%
50%	79%	47%
70%	90%	67%

We can see that the LR+ of 3.75 has a modest influence on our judgement. The presence of olfactory hallucinations noticeably increases the probability that the cause of the patient's altered consciousness is due to seizures. Granted, not a huge amount, despite the high specificity, but definitely noticeable. On the other hand, with the LR- of 0.885 the absence of olfactory hallucinations hardly alters our Prior Probability at all.

These results are consistent with "common wisdom" of Likelihood Ratios. An LR equal to 1.0 is useless, the absence of the symptoms does not alter the probability. A scale for interpreting LR+ suggests that an LR+ of 1 to 3.2 is "Not worth more than a bare mention;" LR+ of 3.2 to 10 is "Substantial;" LR+ of 10 to 100 is "Strong;" and LR+ >100 is "Decisive." Certainly the Posterior probability increases noticeably if the hallucinations are present but in no case do they alter our judgement of what we initially believed. We also see that the presence of hallucinations has a larger effect when the Prior is in the mid-range. This is another common sense feature of Bayesian inference. The less certain we are, the more useful is additional information.

Example 2. Moderate Specificity and Sensitivity

Let's look at another example, involving Parkinson's disease, that involves slightly lower specificity but much higher sensitivity. The difference between these two first tables illustrates the impact of the higher sensitivity.

A 79 year old woman presents with left hand tremor. You notice that she has a masked face. The question in this example is, what is the influence of the masked face on the probability that this patient with tremor has Parkinson's Disease. For purposes of the illustration, I will estimate that masked facies have a specificity of 80% and a sensitivity of 90% for an experienced clinician. With this data we calculate that LR+ = 4.5 and LR- = 0.125. Lets set up the same table as for the first example.

Prior Probability	With Masked Face	Without Masked Face
10%	33%	1%
30%	66%	5%
50%	82%	12%
70%	91%	23%

What can we learn from this? First, the LR+ has a higher value due to the high sensitivity despite the lower specificity. Second, that the LR+ of 4.5 has a significant effect on the Prior, similar to the first example. And again we see larger effects at 30% and 50% Prior. But this time, with the LR- of 0.125, the absence of the finding really matters. For nearly all Priors, there is enough influence of the absence of masked face that we have to seriously consider alternative diagnoses. The higher sensitivity has a major impact.

Example 3. High Sensitivity and Specificity

One more example, from the field of ischemic stroke, using the high Sensitivity and Specificity of Diffusion-Weighted MRI (DWI).

A 57 year old man presents with sudden left sided weakness and you send him for DWI. The question is how strongly the DWI will affect the probability that he has a stroke. From data that we generated at Stony Brook, the Specificity of DWI is 92% and Sensitivity is 96% within 6 hours of symptom onset, yielding remarkable values of LR+ = 12 and LR- = 0.04. Back to the table.

Prior Probability	DWI Positive	DWI Negative
10%	57%	0%
30%	84%	2%
50%	92%	4%
70%	97%	9%

These are really pretty amazing results and highlight the very high sensitivity and specificity of DWI in stroke. No matter what your Prior estimate, you must seriously consider the diagnosis of stroke when the DWI is positive. Similarly, if the DWI does not show evidence of stroke, no matter what you thought before the MRI, you have to give earnest thought to what else it might be. Of course that includes TIA, so you have to be careful.

For comparison, the non-contrast head CT has a sensitivity of 27% within the first 6 hours and I'll estimate the specificity at about 80% so that the LR+ is only 1.35 and the LR- is 0.91. With both values so close to 1.0 you can see why we say that the initial head CT in ischemic stroke is to "rule out hemorrhages and tumors" and not to detect the stroke. DWI was a game changer in the diagnosis of acute stroke and you can see why. It is important to note how the quantitative aspects of this analysis correlate with and help explain our clinical experience.

Summary of the Three Examples and Introducing Two Mnemonic Aids

Let's take a step back and review what we have learned. First, tests are more useful the less certain we are about whether a diagnosis is present or not. Bigger effects are seen the closer we get to a "toss-up."

Secondly, the further a Likelihood Ratio is from 1.0, the more useful it is. Thirdly, Sensitivity and Specificity are both important but have different effects. Tests with high Sensitivity have a major impact when the test is negative. Tests with high Specificity have greater impact when the test is positive. These observations are summarized in the two mnemonic aids, SpPIn and SnNOut.

SpPIn reminds you that in a test with high specificity (Sp), a positive result (P) rules In the diagnosis while SnNOut reminds you that in a test with high sensitivity (Sn), a negative result (N) rules Out the diagnosis. Of course, we never actually rule out a diagnosis but you get the idea. Despite theoretical objections to these rules, I find them reasonably useful in practice as first approximations. I mostly use them to verify and understand what I estimate using Bayes' theorem and Fagan's nomogram based on the Likelihood Ratios.

I hope it is clear that even though these three examples used neurologic patients, everything that we learned from the examples applies to every field of medicine, not just Neurology.

Combining Bayesian Inference with The Universe

In this next section we will explore how combining Bayesian inference and The Universe can help clarify the logic of the diagnostic process, progressively moving toward more complicated scenarios.

Example. Is the Leg Weakness Due to MS or Stroke? Ask a Question!

Let's explore the patient with leg weakness who we said might have a stroke or MS. We used relative incidence of the two diseases to establish a Prior probability for MS. But, now I will allow you to ask me one question before answering. What would your question be? Neurology residents always ask the same question while students and non-Neuro residents usually, but don't always, ask this question. The most useful question is "How old is the patient?" Why? Because, if the patient is 18 years old, it is much more likely to be MS than if the patient is older. But if the patient is 80, stroke is much more likely than in a younger patient. That is intuitively correct but does youth mean that the diagnosis of MS is more likely than stroke? Let's run some calculations and see what happens.

Roughly 90% of MS begins before the age of 40, so instead of 40 per 100,000 patient-years we should use 36. Since 14% of strokes occur in people under the age of 40, if the patient was younger the stroke incidence is not 800 but only 112. Therefore, if the patient is under age 40, then instead of a probability of 40/840, or 5%, the probability would be 36/148, or 24%. Above the age of 40, the relative incidence of MS to stroke is less than 1%. The relative proportions of The Universe definitely change by knowing the patient's age but the incidence of stroke remains higher than that of MS even under the age of 40. Stroke is just that much more common. This is a good example of why it helps to verify your intuitive reasoning with the actual calculation.

Example. Does It Matter if a Patient with Polyuria also has Dysuria?
In our next example, we leave Neurology to consider polyuria. The point of this example is to see how simplifying The Universe can be very useful.

Polyuria has a very broad and complex differential, including use of diuretics, diabetes mellitus (DM), diabetes insipidus, nephrogenic polyuria, primary polyuria, polydipsia and many others. The most common cause for a patient presenting to the ED or their primary doctor with polyuria, however, is a urinary tract infection (UTI). The diagnostic work-up for UTI is relatively straightforward, readily available and inexpensive. Actually, the same is true for DM but the rest of the workup for the differential is complex, to say the least.

So how should we handle this situation? Do we create a multi-compartment Universe and slog our way through? I would recommend not doing that as the full work-up is expensive and time consuming. A reasonable approach would be to divide The Universe in 3 parts, UTI, DM and Other. Rather than focusing on the lab evaluations, for this example, I would like to focus on the presence of the symptom of dysuria, that is pain or discomfort on urination, as the first test. From the literature, in patients with polyuria, dysuria has a sensitivity of 96% with a specificity of 69% for UTI. Therefore, LR+ = 3.1 and LR- = 0.057. If we start with a Prior probability for UTI in our patient with polyuria of 50% using incidence estimates, then the presence of dysuria increases the Posterior probability to 76%, but the absence of dysuria reduces the probability to only 6%. Of course, it isn't only the probability of UTI that changes but the categories of DM and Other will decrease or increase proportionately in response to the presence of this simple, inexpensive and readily available "test." This is a good example of SnNOut since the high sensitivity (and low LR-) make the absence of the symptom a powerful result.

How to Work with A Multi-compartment Universe

What happens when we need to include many compartments? For example, we saw that unexplained loss of consciousness should include syncope, cardiovascular, TIA and epileptic categories as well as other. I assure you that it is possible to proceed quantitatively if you wanted to but that is rarely done. However, the logic remains the same and is, if anything, even more useful.

The Universe is 100%. I often explore the differential for this very common problem with students and residents after hearing their presentation but before we go see the patient together. "OK, so these are the four working diagnoses and we'll add "Other" so that the Universe is 100% and we stay alert to other possibilities. The task is to allocate the total probability among categories just like before but now the 100% is divided into five categories. Again, we each express our independent estimates aloud. Then we go in and speak with the patient and examine them. After we leave the room we discuss what additional information we learned. Then we repeat the above exercise to partition the probabilities into five categories. Maybe we drop one because the mini-ROS was entirely negative. Maybe we add a new possibility. Maybe we didn't learn anything new and the results are unchanged. However, one thing that always changes, if we do such an exercise, is our long-term understanding of diseases and medical reasoning. We all come out better at differential diagnosis and we come away with a very strong intuition of how increasing or decreasing the probability of one diagnosis alters the probabilities of the other diagnoses. I strongly encourage you to try it. In fact, I urge you to make a habit of it.

Concatenating Test Results, the First Posterior is the Next Prior

The following example illustrates the power of Bayesian inference when more than one test is available. The example shows how easy it is to combine the results of two, or even more, tests to vastly improve the accuracy of your probability estimates. Finally, we are approaching the diagnostic process of the real world. At the end of the example, we will also discuss how to decide on the sequence for running tests when more than one test is available.

We saw above that you can use the relative incidence of 15-20% to estimate the probability that an unseen patient with stroke in the ED has an ICH. That's fine but not at all realistic because there are two excellent tests that are readily available in the ED. One is the CT scan and the other is the question of whether the patient has a severe and unusual headache. In this example, we will explore each test independently as well as illustrate how we can use BOTH tests to estimate a better Posterior probability.

Assume that the ED attending tells us that the patient has a severe and unusual headache. How does that change our estimate of the probability that the stroke is hemorrhagic?

Let's use a Prior of 17.5%, midway between 15% and 20%. Based on available literature, 70% of patients with hemorrhagic stroke but only 10% of patients with ischemic stroke have a "severe and unusual headache." So the sensitivity of severe and unusual headache in hemorrhagic stroke is 0.70, the specificity is 0.835, and LR+ = 4.3. Using Fagan's nomogram, with a prior of 17.5%, and LR+ of 4.3, the presence of a severe and unusual headache increases the Posterior probability from the original 17.5% to 47%.

There are other clinical signs that favor ICH as well such as severe hypertension, altered level of consciousness and evidence of increased sympathetic tone. But for now, let's just work with the headache and a CT scan.

Let's do the same analysis with the head CT. The non-contrast head CT scan has a sensitivity of about 98% for hemorrhagic stroke in a patient who presents within 6 hours of symptom onset, although less after 6 hours. The specificity is about 95%. Therefore, LR+ = 19.6. So a positive head CT with the appearance of an ICH increases the Posterior probability from 17.5% to 80%. What? Only 80%? Surprised, aren't you? With those very high sensitivity, specificity and LR+, you would naturally expect a much higher Posterior probability. Just like with the MS case above, this demonstrates why quantifying your estimates can provide important reality checks.

But wait a minute! What if I knew that the patient had a severe and unusual headache before I sent him for the CT scan? Ah-ha! Great question! We can concatenate results with Bayesian logic. You can use ALL of the information together, you do not have to interpret each test independently. That is intuitive to you as a clinician and illustrates again that clinicians are natural Bayesians. Put explicitly, when you run two tests in a row, the Posterior Probability of the first test becomes the Prior Probability of the second test. So let's make use of the headache and then the CT and see what we get.

The Sensitivity, Specificity and LR+ for the headache and CT scan individually are the same of course. What changes is only the Prior for the CT. The unusual headache increased the Prior increases from 17.5% to 47%. With that information taken into account, the positive CT scan moves the Posterior probability to over 95%. That's more like it! This is the kind of confidence that we expected.

But notice one thing, please. The answer is still not 100%. So, if the patient also tells you that for 2 months prior to the onset of severe and unusual headache, they had been having progressive right sided weakness, some confusion and difficulty with language, a mild intermittent morning headache, 15 pounds of weight loss and a new persistent blood-tinged cough after smoking a pack of cigarettes a day for the last 50 years, please promise me that you will consider the possibility that the apparent hemorrhage is actually a metastatic lung tumor. OK?

The sequence of which tests to use first when multiple tests are available is usually obvious if you think about it. The key determining factor is patient safety. You also need to consider the availability of the test, the time and convenience involved in running the test as well as the LR±. Unfortunately, failure to explicitly review these factors often leads to unnecessary risk and patient complications, as well as expense, non-diagnostic results and delays in diagnosis. Any useful tests that can be obtained from the history and physical are a no-brainer. Get the data! As for the rest, in the next chapter, we will take a detailed look at how diagnostic tests interact with treatment decisions. Treatment efficacy and risk, the risk of further testing and patient values will all be considered. Minimizing risk is a key guiding principle.

The mini-ROS

In the last section of this chapter I would like to introduce the clinical tool that I use heavily to help integrate Bayesian hypothesis testing, The Universe with multiple hypotheses and real world clinical diagnosis. I think of this as the mini- Review of Systems or mini-ROS. This mind set changes the nature of the review of systems in a profound way. Instead of being a list of symptoms that you need to review with your patients to complete your note, the mini-ROS becomes a series of powerful tests that you use to evaluate your differential hypotheses. Each disease has a mini-ROS associated with it that you use to test your hypothesis. Depending on how many "Yes" or "No" answers you get, as well as the specificity and sensitivity of each question in the mini-ROS, you increase or decrease the probability of each disease in your differential.

Example. Mini-ROS for Anginal Chest Pain

There is a mini-ROS for virtually every disease that encapsulates the symptoms that are or are not associated with that disease, especially upon presentation. Here is a mini-ROS that you might use to explore the possibility of angina in a patient presenting with chest pain. Note that for some questions a positive responses increases the probability of angina and for some questions a positive response reduces the probability.

Increases Probability

Is the pain pressure-like, as if someone is sitting on your chest?
Does the pain reach up to your neck or left shoulder?
Does the pain increase with exercise?
Does the pain decrease with rest?
Do you have nausea with the pain?
Do you feel short of breath with the pain?
Has anyone in your family had an early heart attack or stroke?
Have you ever had other problems with your heart?
Do you have diabetes or high cholesterol?
Do you smoke?

Decreases Probability

Can you reproduce your pain by pushing on your chest?
Can you reproduce your pain with a deep breath?
Does the pain come when you eat?
Is the pain relieved by burping?
Have you ever been diagnosed with a hiatal hernia?

Make a hypothesis, test a hypothesis. Each positive response to the first group and each negative response to the second groups increases the probability that the patient's chest pain is from angina. The results concatenate. Some tests have higher sensitivity and/or specificity; knowing how to ask the questions can improve both. Scales have been created for use by ED and family physicians, and cardiologists, by quantifying this approach. From the responses, you calculate a probability that the pain is anginal. And now, after reading this chapter, you know where these scales come from. The calculated points for each symptom come from regression analysis.

Example. Combining Multi-Compartment Universe with mini-ROS
Let's consider the common problem of unexplained LOC in a bit more detail to illustrate how we can combine all of the concepts we have been discussing. A patient presents with multiple episodes of brief, unexplained unconsciousness. Our differential is syncope, cardiac, TIA, seizure and other. The Universe is 100%. We know that seizure and TIA are less common than syncope or cardiac so we could assign them Prior Probabilities of about 10% each. The four explicit entities make up the large majority of cases, so we also might assign 10% to Other. Let's go 40% syncope and 30% cardiac, with no information from the patient, this is all based on incidence data.

Now we apply our mini-ROS as tests to increase or decrease the Posterior Probabilities. Here are some key questions (there are many others) that will help. Syncope virtually always occurs with the patient in the upright position, standing or sitting upright, so if the patient has events while lying down, the probability of syncope falls to less than 5% (and the others increase proportionately). But if the patient has symptoms of orthostatic dizziness, then syncope becomes much more likely. If the patient experienced palpitations before the LOC or has a prior history of heart disease, cardiac becomes more likely since palpitations are reasonably specific. If palpitations were not present, however, our probabilities do not change very much because palpitations have only a modest sensitivity. If the patient has been experiencing any focal neurologic deficits either in the past or prior to the LOC, then the probability of TIA and seizure increase considerably (and cardiac and syncope become much less likely). LOC with TIA would almost certainly have to involve the brainstem so focal brainstem symptoms such as diplopia prior to onset of other symptoms would carry high specificity and strongly increase that probability. (Vertigo can occur with any of the causes and so has poor specificity.) The mini-ROS for epilepsy has reasonably good specificity. So if there have been clonic limb or face movements, or visual, auditory or olfactory hallucinations, or *déjà vu*, then the Probability of seizure as the cause of LOC climbs dramatically. The more seizure symptoms are present, the higher the probability since the test results can concatenate. If there have been no seizure symptoms then its probability decreases well below 10% although it never quite disappears. But other entities become more likely.

Get the idea? We didn't need to use Fagan's nomogram for this differential. The qualitative reasoning and logic was perfectly adequate.

One Last Parting Recommendation and Example

Don't try to fit a round peg into a square hole! You have to learn when the diagnosis fits and when it doesn't. We all want to find an answer and the diagnostic process often develops a momentum around a particular diagnosis. Unfortunately, when that happens, we tend to ignore information which is contrary to the diagnosis, whether clinical or lab. We risk developing "blinders" and seeing only straight ahead, confirming what we think we know when we should, instead, stop and reassess the data and our interpretations.

A VERY common example. It may be virtually impossible to separate common migraine from sinusitis on clinical grounds. The best answer I know is from the history. If the patient has disgusting discharge from his nose and down his throat, then it is sinusitis. But it may be sinusitis even without that (the sensitivity is good if you ask correctly but not better than 80%). So clinicians often order a low radiation CT scan of the sinuses to detect the sinusitis. CT has a sensitivity of 95% and specificity of 92% for sinusitis. So the LR+ is 12 and LR- is 0.05. Let's assume 50/50 Prior probability. A negative CT scan reduces the probability of sinusitis from 50% to 5%. Unfortunately, in many, many cases, the clinician continues to treat for sinusitis. Would you? I would not if I were the treating physician. Especially if they did not have disgusting drainage (concatenating tests). And if they DID have disgusting drainage, I would have treated without the CT scan since migraine virtually never causes disgusting drainage.

Clearly, we have now reached the real world of clinical diagnosis. I hope that the LOGIC of this approach has been made clear and that we have not lost the forest for the trees. Nothing needs to be memorized. It's an approach, your attitude, that matters, supported by a few basic and universally applicable tools.

What Are the Take-away Lessons of this Chapter?

1. The greatest value of Bayesian inference is thinking about diagnosis as a series of hypotheses that must be tested.
2. The Universe is a valuable concept for organizing your thoughts.
3. You will be able to estimate Prior probabilities intuitively very early in your career. You can also rely on incidence data to estimate a Prior, if available.
4. Tests with the largest LR+ or smallest LR- are the most useful but expense, availability and timeliness, as well as patient risk and comfort, must be taken into consideration when choosing tests. In most cases, a detailed history, including the use of mini-ROS's, are the obvious first choice.
5. While quantification is often not necessary, it is possible, and at times it can yield surprising results that may change your perspective on testing strategies.
6. Bayesian estimates are actually distributions of probabilities.
7. Test results can and should be concatenated. You add all of your information together to obtain your estimates of the probability that a disease is present.

Integrating Differential Diagnosis with Treatment

Differential diagnosis is not just about probabilities. When you prioritize your list of diagnoses, the order is emphatically not sorted simply by probability. Other important factors may take precedence. For example, most of us would prefer to diagnose a treatable condition than an untreatable one. I sometimes say that missing a B12 deficiency or hypothyroidism is a sin because they are SO easy to treat and can have such severe consequences if left untreated. Differential diagnosis is not performed in isolation. It is done for the sake of a real person who is sick and is dependent upon us for help. Differential diagnosis is merely a first step on the way to caring for the patient and must be integrated into the rest of our care. In particular, we must decide when we have enough information to make the necessary therapeutic decisions. Are we confident of our diagnoses? Do we have enough information or do we need more tests? That's why the Bayesian estimates and distributions are so valuable in differential diagnosis. They lead seamlessly to decision making.

And with that understanding we are ready to move on to the next chapter on therapeutic decisions. In that chapter, we will merge the diagnostic process with the process of therapeutic decision making. Some of the interactions between the two are obvious but some are deep and subtle, reaching to the heart of our roles as doctors.

Chapter 5. Therapeutic Decisions

Introduction

The goal of this chapter is to build a structure for helping you make therapeutic decisions.

This chapter stands out in several ways. My mentor Dr. Fritz Dreifuss once said, "The essential role of a doctor is to make decisions." This same sentiment is implicit in Osler's comment about probability and uncertainty. Thus, this chapter is at the cognitive center of this book. Secondly, because decision making is multi-dimensional, the chapter has been particularly challenging to write clearly and logically. For that reason, I will resort to even more transparency than usual. Specifically, you will notice:

Increased use of outline with clearly defined sub-sections

Progressing with many small steps using examples to derive concepts and to reduce the density of the reading

Reflecting on our progress frequently.

The challenge for all of us, but especially for beginning physicians, is how to organize the sophisticated science and art of decision making into a process that is rigorous, flexible, compassionate and practical. The process must be robust enough to handle the complexity, and to include patient specific goals and values, while being practical enough to fit into our busy routines.

The Neural Basis of Decision Making

The cognitive aspects of the process have interested me since I had to give a neuroscience lecture to Stony Brook medical students in 1982. I chose then to begin with a whimsical analogy which has remained with me ever since.

Imagine that there is a car filled with five Stony Brook medical students heading north on the New York Thruway to a day of skiing at Butternut in Massachusetts. It's early in the morning and things are going along fine until the driver sees a sign that says, "Rest Stop, Two Miles." He asks aloud, "Shall we stop at the Rest Stop?"

Now imagine what goes on in the minds of the five students as they ponder this question. Are they early for the mountain opening or are they running late? Does anyone have to use the rest room? Is anyone hungry? How far to the next Rest Stop? Does anyone in the back have motion sickness and wants to switch to the front seat? Does anyone want to change seats to get away from someone or maybe to get closer to someone? So many things to consider!

The driver then sees the sign "Rest Stop, One Mile." He moves over to the right lane to prepare for a last second decision and says, "Come on guys. Are we stopping or not?"

Here's the point. No matter how many influences there are on this decision, there are only two possible choices. Either they pull off and stop or they continue. There are no other possibilities.

This analogy captures essential features of our brain's process of decision making. It is capable of using a huge number of factors to make a decision but, all of this get's fed into a group of neurons in our dorsolateral pre-frontal cortex that are known as Go - NoGo neurons. We can prepare very complex, multi-faceted plans but, in the end, we must decide if, and when, to execute that plan. Either we execute the plan or we do not.

This All-or-None feature of our brain is embedded in our medical decision making. You might object that medical decisions are complex, that our plans can have many pieces and that there are many paths that we might follow to complete the plan. I would agree with those statements but respond that assembling the plan, evaluating the conditions for if and when to execute it, as well as how to modify it as the patient's course unfolds, all can be explained as a process of bifurcating Yes/No decisions.

As an example let's focus on a small subset of factors involved in the decision of whether or not to give TNK to a patient with an acute stroke.

1. Is this a stroke?
2. Is it safe for this patient to receive TNK?
3. Are there modifiable factors such as hypertension that should delay the use of TNK until brought under control?

Let's assume that your medical center's Stroke Program is very protocol driven and has an explicit set of Inclusion/Exclusion Criteria for TNK as well as a detailed TNK Order Set. As you review the patient's eligibility, you can view the Inclusion criteria as a series of Yes or No decisions or the whole set of Inclusion criteria as one Yes or No decision. It doesn't matter, you see. Either way it comes to Yes or No. The same is true of the Exclusion Criteria.

Assume you decide to proceed with thrombolysis. You turn to the Order Set. It is an explicit set of orders which either have to be checked to be ordered or must be completed with specific input to make the order active. Again, whether you view the individual orders as the decision points or whether to activate the entire order set as a single decision, you are facing Yes or No decisions.

In other words, you can view each criteria or order as a Yes/No decision or you can choose to make the bundle the Yes/No decision point. Either way, the decision is Yes or No. Logically, you are dealing with IF, THEN decisions. If you choose to focus on the individual, discrete decisions then you are saying:
IF {condition is met}, THEN {execute action};
but if you focus on the bundle, then you are saying:
IF {condition set is met}, THEN {execute set of actions}.

OK? With these considerations in mind, let's begin to create the therapeutic decision making structure described above. We will proceed step by step, from the simplest possible scenario to full clinical complexity, including patient preferences.

Introducing Decision Thresholds
Medical decisions involve two thresholds, the Treatment Threshold and the Testing Threshold. These two thresholds divide the status of therapeutic decisions into three possibilities:
1. One possibility is that your estimate of the probability of a disease in a patient is high enough that you are above the Treatment Threshold and are ready to begin treating the patient.
2. Another possibility is that your estimate of the disease probability in your patient is so low that you are below the testing threshold and are not going to pursue the diagnosis any further, at least for now.
3. The third possibility is that you are in between the two thresholds, not ready to treat but not ready to ignore the diagnosis. You haven't "made up your mind."

This is the basis of the structure that we want to develop. The rest of this chapter will expand on these two thresholds and three possible states to develop that structure in detail.

Using this structure requires two steps. First you have to set your Treatment and Testing Thresholds. Secondly, you have to evaluate the probability of the disease in your patient and determine if the probability crosses either threshold.

These thresholds are not fixed numbers that we choose based on statistics (like a "95% confidence limit"). Rather, they are set for each patient individually using medical judgement based on clinical factors. Setting the thresholds involve judgements that you must make based on factors that characterize your patient, the disease of interest, treatment efficacy and risk, testing accuracy and risk, and the capabilities of your medical center. Determining whether you have crossed either threshold, as you might guess, involves probability estimates of the type that we considered in the last chapter.

From here on we will use Examples to develop our concepts and the structure we seek. Although the initial examples may seem trivial, follow carefully because the later examples certainly will not be.

Example #1.
Diagnosis is Certain
Treatment Has Benefit and No Cost
Treatment Threshold Always Reached
No Role for Testing

Assume that there is a patient who is known to have a certain disease which has a natural history of 50% mortality in one year. Assume also that there is a treatment that reduces mortality from 50% for untreated patients to 20% with treatment. Assume finally that there are no side effects from this treatment. We define the variable "Benefit" for a patient who actually has the disease, as the the net sum of all probable benefits minus the net sum of all probable costs related to treatment. Since there is no cost in this case, we can calculate the net benefit as, Benefit = (50% - 20%) - 0% = 30%.

There is no question here. We know the patient has the disease and we know the treatment has a 30% net benefit without any side effects. Obviously, any patient with this disease should receive the treatment. Furthermore, even if we only suspect that the patient has the disease, they still should be treated because there is no cost to treatment. There is no need for testing since there are no significant side effects if we treat patients who do not actually have the disease.

New Concept Introduced:
Net Benefit

Example #2.
Diagnosis Is Not Certain
Treatment With Benefit But Also Cost in the Same Units as Benefit
Treatment Threshold Relevant Since Treating Healthy Patients Risks Harm
Testing Threshold Not Relevant in Absence of Useful Diagnostic Tests

Now let's assume that we are treating a patient in whom we are not certain that they have the disease. Furthermore, new research has demonstrated that the 20% of patients who die despite the treatment are actually in two groups. Ten percent of the patients die because of disease progression but the other 10% die due to side effects of the treatment. This is obviously a more complicated situation because there is potential to do harm if we treat patients without the disease. For the moment, assume that there are no useful diagnostic tests.

Now we do have a question. At what probability that the patient has the disease should you recommend treatment, given the net benefit of 30% mortality reduction in patients with the disease and 10% risk of mortality in patients without the disease?

We have benefits and costs, up sides and down sides. This is much more realistic. Recall that we defined "Benefit" as the net benefit minus the net cost for treating patients with the disease. When the diagnosis is uncertain, we may end up treating some patients who do not have the disease. They experience no treatment benefit but they are at risk for treatment-related side effects. We define "Cost" as the net cost of all probable side effects experienced by <u>treated patients without the disease</u>. In this example, we limit ourselves to the simplified situation where Benefit and Cost are in the same units, namely mortality. Benefit is still 30%, but now Cost is 10%. (The terms "Cost" and "Harm" will be used synonymously.) We will deal with diagnostic tests in the next example.

First let's look at the extremes. If the patient had a 90% probability of the disease, would you treat? Well, if there were 100 patients with a 90% probability who were treated, 90 patients with the disease would receive the net benefit of 30%, so 27 lives would be saved. On the other hand, the 10% without the disease would have been exposed to the 10% risk of death so that 1 additional patient would have died. The overall improvement to treating this population with 90% disease probability would be 26 lives saved, so treatment would be indicated.

Towards the opposite extreme, if the patient had a 10% probability of the disease, would you treat? Well, if there were 100 patients with a

10% probability who were treated, 10 patients with the disease would receive the net benefit of 30%, so 3 lives would be saved. On the other hand, the 90% without the disease would have been exposed to the 10% risk of death so that 9 additional patients would have died. The overall affect of treating this population with 10% disease probability would be an additional 6 lives lost, so treatment certainly would not be indicated.

OK, then. The question, of course, is at what probability of disease for a particular patient would you treat? It can be shown that the answer is contained in the following simple equation based on the Benefit for patients with the disease and the Cost to patients without the disease. We will call this probability the "Treatment Threshold," where:

$$Treatment\ Threshold = \frac{1}{\left(1 + \dfrac{Benefit}{Cost}\right)}$$

The central idea of the Treatment Threshold is that at that probability a fair and honest clinician would be indifferent to the choice of treatment or not. Since in this case, Benefit is 30% and Cost is 10%, the Benefit/Cost Ratio is 3 and the Treatment Threshold is 1/4, or 25%. If the probability of the disease in a patient is estimated to be above 25%, then treatment should be recommended but not if the probability is below the 25% Treatment Threshold.

This example is still relatively straightforward but we have introduced diagnostic uncertainty and introduced the useful concepts of Benefit, Cost or Harm, and the Treatment Threshold which is calculated from the Benefit and Cost.

New Concepts Introduced:
Risk of Harm with Treatment
Uncertainty of Diagnosis, No Further Testing Available
Explicit Calculation of Treatment Threshold Based on Benefit/Cost Ratio

Example #3
Diagnosis Is Not Certain
Treatment With Benefit and Cost in Same Units
Treatment Threshold Is Relevant
Diagnostic Test with a Risk of Harm in Same Units,, so a Testing Threshold will be Needed

Now lets make the example still more realistic. In addition to diagnostic uncertainty and the potential for harm with treatment, let us assume that there is a test that can help us alter the probability that the patient has the disease using exactly the same testing principles of the last chapter but with one important additional feature. The test carries risk. For the moment, to maintain simplicity of calculations, we will assume that the risk can be expressed in the same units as the Benefit and Cost, namely that there is a risk of mortality. Don't be shocked! Think about organ biopsies or even nodal ablation for atrial fibrillation. Trust me, they carry small but very real risks, including mortality. Even the genetic blood test for Huntington's Disease carries a risk of suicide. Later on, we will address how to compare Benefits, Costs and Side Effects that differ.

Let's assume that we have access to a diagnostic test with LR+ of 4 and LR- of 0.3, but which carries a 2% risk of mortality. If we test everyone, the net Benefit, including the 2% risk of testing, would fall from 30% to 28%, and the net Cost would increase to 12% mortality. So, would you administer the test to everyone? If not, how do you decide when to use the test? This is a very important example for us to think through. You can see why we need structure for our decisions. Tranquilo. Paso a paso.

Primum non nocere. First, do no harm. Personally, I find that a very complex principle to implement in practice. However, I believe with all my heart that you should never run an <u>unnecessary</u> risk. Never. If the risk isn't useful, there is no justification for allowing that risk to enter the clinical scenario. In this case, testing involves a 2% risk of death. That is not small. You can verify that including the 2% testing mortality rate in Benefit and Cost as above increases the Treatment Threshold from 25% to 30%. But even if the cost was smaller, the principle would remain that you should only do the test if it is useful. Practically speaking, the question is whether we can limit when we use this test with potential harm to avoid unnecessary risk?

We start by using standard Aristotelian deductive logic, not Bayesian inference, statistics or even clinical judgement. The necessary reasoning is a bit complicated so follow closely.

First, assume that our Prior estimate of the disease probability in a patient is greater than the re-calculated Treatment Threshold of 30%. In that case, testing can change our mind about treatment only if it reduces the disease probability to below 30% because of a negative test result. Increasing the probability further doesn't modify our decision. Therefore, with the Prior already above the Treatment Threshold of 30%, it is the negative likelihood ratio, LR-, that is relevant. The test should have a high Sensitivity (SnNOut). On the other hand, if our Prior estimate is below 30%, then the test can change our mind only by increasing the Probability to above the Treatment Threshold due to a positive test result, so the LR+ would be relevant. The test should have a high Specificity (SpPIn).

So when is this test with potential harm useful and when is it not necessary? There are two specific questions that arise from this logic. First, at what Prior Probability of the disease is the value so high that even a negative test result will leave us above the Treatment Threshold? We have an LR- of 0.3. We need to calculate the Prior at which the Post-test Probability will remain above 30% even if the test comes back negative.

The second question is the converse. At what Prior Probability will the Post-test Probability remain so low that even a positive test result will leave us below the Treatment Threshold? That is, with a LR+ of 4, at what Prior will the Post-test Probability remain below 30% even with a positive test result.

We don't want to run any unnecessary, useless risks.

The technique for obtaining the answer to both questions is the same. Use Fagan's nomogram BACKWARDS. That is, instead of putting your straight edge on the Prior (left vertical) and running through the LR± to find the Posterior Probability (right vertical), we will start by putting the straight edge on the Posterior and run through the LR± to find the Prior. Let's look at the two scenarios separately, first with a Prior Probability estimate above 30%, when the LR- is relevant, and then with a Prior estimate below 30%, when the LR+ is relevant.

If your Prior is above 30%, and you run the straight edge from 30% through the LR-, then you will find the Prior which defines the level of Prior which cannot be brought below 30% with the available test. When you do this, you will find that, using the values provided above, if your Prior is above 59%, even a negative test result will leave you with a Post-test Probability above 30% and you would treat. Therefore, if your Prior is greater than 59%, you would not be justified in accepting the 2% risk of mortality and you should not bother with the test. Just go ahead and treat. This defines the Treatment Threshold when a useful test with risk is available.

On the other hand, if your Prior is below 30%, run the straight edge from 30% on the right through the LR+ and you will find the Prior which cannot be brought above 30% even with a positive test result. Using the LR+ of 4, the Post-test Probability will remain below 30% if your Prior is below 10%. So, with a Prior less than 10%, there is no justification for running the mortality risk associated with testing. The test cannot change your mind. Do not run the test. This provides the Testing Threshold when a useful test with risk is available.

To summarize this complicated example, if your Prior is below 10% then do not treat and do not test. If your prior is above 59% then treat without testing. If your Prior is between the Testing Threshold of

10% and Treating Threshold of 59% then it is justified to use the test because it can provide useful information. If the test is positive then you would treat but if the test is negative then you would not. Whether you actually do or do not use the test, however, is a much more complicated matter that we will address shortly.

The following figure illustrates these definitions and principles.

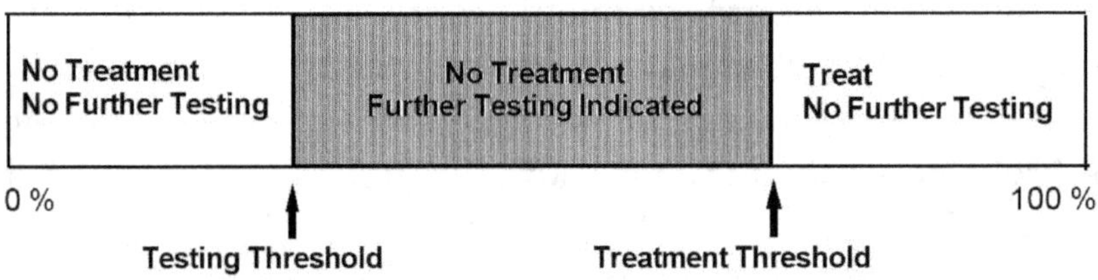

Below the Testing Threshold, there is no test that is sufficiently safe and has the necessary LR+ to increase the patient's probability of disease to the point that we would decide to treat. We should not treat or test any further. Presumably, we would elect to observe the patient clinically over time to see if anything changes to alter the probability. We will re-consider this option later in this chapter.

Above the Treatment Threshold, there is no test that is sufficiently safe and has the necessary LR- to alter our decision to proceed with treatment. We should go ahead and treat without further testing.

Between the two thresholds, we have decided that we want more information. It is our judgement that we do not have sufficient confidence to treat or to stop considering treatment. Fortunately, there is a test with likelihood ratios that are capable of altering our recommendations within this range, either to proceed toward treatment or withhold treatment albeit with risk.

I must confess that I have taken some minor liberties in the threshold calculations for the sake of conceptual clarity in this discussion. For a completely rigorous discussion of the calculations, I recommend that you read Reference 2 which is cited on page 142.

This is as far as we are going to take quantitative decision making. In the rest of the chapter, we will address the many factors that contribute to how you actually use the concepts of Treatment and Testing Thresholds for the care of an individual patient. If all of this has not been sufficiently clear, consider re-reading the chapter thus far and/or looking at the cited references before proceeding.

New Concepts Introduced:
Having Available Tests With Risk of Harm
The Testing Threshold
The Treatment Threshold With Testing Available
Using Fagan's Nomogram Backwards to Identify When Testing Would Run Unnecessary Risk

The next two examples are drawn from my own practice. These two cases taught me to pay attention to these thresholds.

Example #4.
Patient with High Probability of Temporal Arteritis
Treatment with Prednisone
Testing with Temporal Artery Biopsy
Whether or Not to Continue Prednisone with Negative Biopsy

A 68 year old woman who I had treated several years earlier for a non-disabling stroke presented to my clinic at Stony Brook on a Friday afternoon with a new problem. She had been experiencing a variety of visual disturbances involving both eyes with transient scotomata and occasional diplopia for more than 2 weeks. She also had jaw pain on chewing, mild diffuse myalgias and intermittent unusual headaches. She had no known systemic diseases. Her temporal arteries were mildly tender. My working diagnosis was temporal arteritis (Giant Cell Arteritis). I sent her for an ESR and started her on prednisone 60 mg daily. I also set up an appointment in Ophthalmology for a temporal artery biopsy and return visit to see me in 2 weeks. When she returned in two weeks, the ESR had been 126, her symptoms had nearly completely disappeared, she was still taking the prednisone as instructed and her temporal artery biopsy was Negative.

What did I do with the steroids? I continued them of course! But it bothered me that I did so despite the negative biopsy, even though I firmly believed that was the right thing to do. What really bothered me was why I did the relatively invasive TA biopsy and then ignored the negative results.

For the first time in my career I followed the procedure outlined above. Of course it was too late to benefit my patient but it influenced my practice for the next 25 years. Based on all of the clinical information and the ESR of 126, I estimated my Prior as greater than 95% that she had temporal arteritis, let's say 96%. With literature values for temporal artery biopsy of 80% sensitivity and 95% specificity at that time, her LR- was 0.21. So the negative test result left an 83% probability that she had temporal arteritis. Clearly, in retrospect, it was not justified to do the biopsy. I had already seen patients experience a variety of minor complications and even one major complication from temporal artery biopsy. If the result was positive, obviously I would continue treatment. But even when the result was negative I still continued treatment. After working through the numbers, I understood why I continued the steroids but from that day forward, I have been very careful to use deductive logic and Bayesian inference to guide my decisions regarding any test that runs more than trivial risk or cost. I rarely do the actual calculations but I do weigh these factors semi-quantitatively in my decision.

New Concepts Introduced or Emphasized:
With High Prior and Weak LR- Testing May Not Alter Treatment Decision
Avoid Unnecessary Invasive Testing That Cannot Alter Treatment

Example #5.
Patient with Possible Herpes Simplex Encephalitis
Treatment with Acyclovir
Testing with CSF PCR of HSV1
Whether to Await Test Results to Initiate Treatment

The first treatment for Herpes Simplex encephalitis (HSVE) became available in the 1970's, when I was an intern (PGY-1) in Internal Medicine. Acyclovir followed shortly thereafter. These drugs were a miracle as far as I was concerned since they took what was a nearly uniformly fatal disease and saved the majority of patients if the drug was administered promptly. Most patients presented within 24 hours of onset since they were sick as s*** with fever, altered consciousness and status epilepticus. Initially, no specific tests were available to make the diagnosis. There were no specific viral tests for HSV, MRI had been invented but was not in clinical application yet, CT was low resolution and of limited sensitivity and specificity. CSF exam demonstrated a non-specific "hemorrhagic encephalitis."

So the question became, at what Prior level of probability based on the clinical data would you administer vidarabine or acyclovir once it became available in the 1980's? You should immediately think of the equation that we wrote for the Treatment Threshold. The important variable is the Benefit/Cost ratio. We could estimate the Benefit as at least 60% reduction in mortality or severe morbidity with treatment. And the Cost? It is nearly impossible to identify a serious side effect since human metabolism is virtually inert to the effects of these anti-virals. In that case Benefit/Cost becomes nearly infinite because Cost approaches zero. So the Treatment Threshold approaches zero. We would virtually be back to Example #1. Well, what about in this age of available PCR for HSV Type 1? Sorry, no, the logic stays the same. HSVE is a life threatening emergency with time line for successful treatment measured in hours. By the time you do an LP, get the sample to the lab, have the lab run the test and get the results, the damage would have increased severely, even in a modern, well-run hospital. So, at what probability of HSVE do you give the first dose of acyclovir? My answer is that if the diagnosis occurs to you as a realistic possibility, then treat immediately and consider stopping the drug if/when the PCR returns negative and an alternative diagnosis is confirmed.

New Concepts Introduced or Emphasized:
Choosing the Treatment Threshold is Heavily Influenced by the Benefit/Cost Ratio
Test Result Availability Must Match the Rate of Disease Evolution to Be Useful
Bayesian Inference Is Useful Even Without Specific Calculations

Example #6.
Patient with Bell's Palsy
Treatment with Prednisone
Treatment Risk Which Is Different Than Benefit
How to Involve Patient Preferences and Values

Now let's look at a much more complex although fanciful example created by a friend, neurologist, biostatistician, teacher and all around good guy (albeit occasionally devious with his friends), Dr. Michael Glantz. This will allow us to delve into quantitative aspects of patient preferences and values when disease consequences and treatment or testing side effects are not the same.

Let's assume that you are Dr. McCoy on the Starship Enterprise and Spock comes in to your office with suspected Bell's Palsy. Let's also assume that, for Vulcans with Bell's Palsy, there is a 100% chance of permanent facial palsy without treatment, a 50% chance of cure if treated with prednisone, but also a 10% risk of negatively impacting their logic if they are treated. If benefit and cost are considered equal, Benefit = 100% - 50% -10% = 40%; Cost = 10%. Assume there is no useful diagnostic test. So, with permanent facial palsy and loss of logic equally important, the Treatment Threshold would be equal to 1 / (1 + Benefit/Cost) = 1 / (1+0.4/0.1) = 1 / (1+4) = 1/5, or 20%. McCoy feels the diagnosis is 25% probable, which is obviously greater than 20%, and so would recommend treatment, IF Spock gives equal value to facial weakness and loss of logic.

However, since the consequences of treating and not treating are very different, and Vulcans can be very fussy about assumptions, McCoy decides to assess Spock's values regarding the relative impacts of improvement versus harm. Spock says that the benefit of being able raise one eyebrow to convey a knowing and skeptical look is moderately important. But the impact of losing his logic is very high.

We'll offer some suggestions about how to obtain input from your patients shortly but, for now, let's just say that Vulcans are so logical that McCoy simply asks Spock how important each factor is on a 0 to 100% scale, from not important at all to extremely important. That's often all you will need to do for your patients as well.

Spock responds that the one eyebrow thing is pretty important and gives it 50% but logic is everything to a Vulcan and gives that 100%. Should McCoy still recommend treatment?

How does Dr. McCoy utilize Spock's preferences quantitatively? The answer is by adding weights to the benefit and cost in order to obtain a Patient Weighted Benefit (PWB) and Patient Weighted Cost (PWC), where PWB still applies to patients with the disease and PWC applies to patients without the disease.

PWB = *(probability of improvement* x *patient weighted impact of that improvement) - (probability of harm* x *patient weighted impact of that harm)*

PWC = *probability of harm* x *patient weighted impact of that harm*

With those adjustments we can continue to use the same equation that we used previously but now we use PWB/PWC instead of the simple Benefit/Cost. Dr. McCoy would then calculate as follows, under Spock's watchful gaze of course.

The Treatment Threshold equation becomes
Treatment Threshold = 1 / (1 + PWB/PWC)

Given a 50% likelihood of benefit with a 50% patient weighted impact and a 10% likelihood of producing loss of logic with a 100% patient weighted impact,

PWB = (0.5 x 0.5) - (0.1 x 1) = 0.25 - 0.1 = 0.15 , and

PWC = 0.1 x 1.0 = 0.1 .

Using these modified values,

Treatment Threshold = 1 / (1 + 0.15/0.1) = 1 / (1 + 1.5) = 1/2.5 = 40% .

Since this Treatment Threshold is considerably above the estimated 25% probability that the disease is present, Dr. McCoy should not recommend treatment. Poor Spock, losing that eyebrow look. But at least it was his choice based on his own values.

So, basically, that is how we take into account patient and family values and preferences. Of course, not all of our patients are as logical as Spock. We will address the question of how to obtain semi-quantitative preferences from patient and family later in this chapter.

In reality, there is usually more than one benefit and more than one side effect involved in a treatment. Fortunately, it is possible to modify the Treatment Threshold equation simply by calculating the sum of all patient weighted consequences as follows.

Total Patient Weighted Benefit (TPWB) =

$$(PWB_1 + PWB_2 + PWB_3 \ldots) - (PWC_1 + PWC_2 + PWC_3 \ldots)$$

and
Total Patient Weighted Cost (TPWC) = $(PWC_1 + PWC_2 + PWC_3 \ldots)$,

where PWB_i and PWC_i are the individual patient weighted benefits and costs based on probability of occurrence and patient weighted impact in patients with (TPWB) and without (TPWC) the disease, respectively.

Treatment Threshold becomes simply:

Treatment Threshold = 1 / (1 + TPWB/TPWC) .

In practice we rarely if ever run that calculation explicitly. But we DO use it heuristically in our discussions with our patients.

New Concepts Introduced or Emphasized:
How to Calculate the Treatment Threshold With Benefits and Costs That Differ
How to Involve Patient (or Family) Preferences and Values In Your Calculations
How to Address Multiple Benefits and Risks

Transition From Concepts to Practices at the Bedside

All of the basic concepts involved in medical decision making have been introduced at this point. It is time to explore the practical side of this approach and translate these concepts into actions at the bedside.

As a brief transition, let's summarize the primary factors which influence how we choose to set the Treatment and Testing Thresholds. These factors will relate to the Disease, the Treatment, the Test and the Patient. Note that the probability that the disease is present is not altered by any of these considerations. It is what we do that changes.

The Treatment Threshold will move to a lower pre-test probability (so you will treat more people) in so far as:

1. The Disease
    a. has serious potential consequences if untreated

b. has risk of producing serious permanent injury suddenly and without warning

2. Treatment
   a. is effective
   b. has low risk
3. Testing
   a. is inaccurate
   b. has high risk and/or cost
   c. is not available in a timely manner
4. The Patient
   a. expresses high concerns about the disease-specific consequences
   b. is resistant to the costs of further testing

Setting the Testing Threshold is a bit more complicated because, as discussed above, the purpose of testing depends on whether our disease Prior Probability estimate is above or below the Treatment Threshold.

If the Prior is above the Treatment Threshold, then the purpose of testing is to see if the diagnosis is less likely than we believe. This happens only with a negative test result so the relevant likelihood is LR- (SnNOut). Under this scenario, you will move the Testing Threshold to lower Prior values (you will test more people) in so far as the Benefit/Cost ratio for treatment is low and Testing is safe and sensitive. Specifically when:

1. The Disease
   a. has milder potential consequences if untreated
   b. is unlikely to produce serious permanent injury suddenly and without warning
2. Treatment
   a. is less effective
   b. has high risk
3. Testing
   a. has high Sensitivity
   b. has low risk and cost

c. is available in a timely manner

4. The Patient
    a. expresses high concerns about the treatment-specific side effects
    b. is tolerant of the costs of further testing

However, if the Prior estimate of disease probability is <u>below</u> the Treatment Threshold, then the test can change our mind only by increasing the Probability to above the Treatment Threshold with a positive test result, so the LR+ would be relevant. The test should have a high Specificity (SpPIn). Since the Testing Threshold is the Probability below which you will choose not to test, the Testing Threshold will move to lower Prior values (you will test more people) in so far as the Benefit/Cost ratio of treatment is high and testing is safe and specific. That is, when:

1. The Disease
    a. has serious potential consequences if untreated
    b. is more likely to produce serious permanent injury suddenly and without warning
2. Treatment
    a. is effective
    b. has low risk
3. Testing
    a. has high Specificity
    b. has low risk and cost
    c. is available in a timely manner
4. The Patient
    a. expresses high concerns about the disease-specific consequences
    b. is tolerant of the costs of further testing

Sorry if that seems complicated, but it is. That's why structured analysis is useful.

<u>Clinical Factors Which Affect the Benefit/Cost Ratio and Thresholds</u>

Now we are ready to explore the various clinical factors that contribute to where we set the Treatment and Testing Thresholds.

As we do this, it will also become clear how closely differential diagnosis and treatment decisions are related. In most patients, the two proceed in parallel simultaneously.

Ultimately, both thresholds are heavily influenced by the Benefit/Cost ratio. As Benefit decreases or Cost increases, the ratio decreases. Both thresholds increase. Fewer patients are treated while the number tested depends on the relative change of the two thresholds. The discussion that follows is a discussion of clinical factors which alter the benefits of treating the disease as well as the costs of additional testing and the treatment itself. The factors affecting Benefit/Cost divide into three major categories: patient specific, disease specific and medical center specific.

Patient Specific Factors Affecting the Benefit/Cost Ratio and Thresholds

Patient specific factors arise both from the medical status of the patient and from the preferences of the patient and family.

The medical status of the patient reflects their pre-morbid health and functional status, as well as how the current disease has altered their health thus far. The rapidity with which the disease is progressing is of critical importance. We will address how the characteristics of the disease directly affect thresholds in the next section. Here our emphasis is on how the disease has altered the patient. In particular, how well the patient is able to tolerate the course of treatment, including necessary additional tests. Disease states often exert a metabolic toll on the patient that lessens their resilience. They also may introduce psychological burdens that further reduce the patient's ability to tolerate treatment related side effects. It is well-known that the metabolic and psychological factors interact heavily. The metabolic changes related to cancer and inflammatory diseases clearly increase the risk of apathy, anorexia and depression. In turn, depression reduces food intake, worsening the catabolic state and there may be other unproven effects on the immune and other systems. Patients in advanced disease stages often respond less well to treatment and have decreased tolerance for treatment-related toxicity. These same factors also influence the patient's capacity for rehabilitation through increased fatigue and decreased motivation. Finally, other pre-existing diseases may reduce the patient's life expectancy. All of these factors reduce the potential benefit of treatment and increase the cost of both treatment and testing.

When there is diagnostic uncertainty, the lowered Benefit/Cost ratio raises the Treatment Threshold to a higher probability. Even if the diagnosis has been well established, the reduced Benefit and increased Costs have a direct impact on treatment decisions, possibly to the point that the Cost may exceed the Benefit.

The degree of family support is an important factor affecting patient tolerance for treatment-related complications as well as maintaining motivation for recovery in rehab. That is one more reason that the family should be involved in helping establish patient preferences.

Accounting for Patient Preferences

In the Example involving Spock, we saw how to incorporate patient values in the Threshold calculations. However, humans are not as logical as Vulcans. So how do we obtain information about preferences and values from our patients in the real world?

Dr. McCoy used a simple linear scale to obtain Spock's valuation of each consequence independently. You can ask the patient to indicate the importance of each consequence using a simple 0 - 10 scale, presented either verbally or visually as a horizontal number line. A useful visual way of presenting that is with a thermometer-looking picture with the scale of 0 at the bottom and either 10 or 100% at the top. Just have the patient point where on the scale their value lies. If 10 seems too difficult, use 0 - 5 and each number becomes 20%. That is 3 out of 5 indicates a 60% impact.

Sometimes it is easier to ask the patient to compare the two outcomes directly to obtain a relative weighting, eg - getting rid of these headaches would be twice as important as having occasional facial twitching during the day. Personally, I think people have an easier time when you use money. So if the patient tells me that Consequence A is worse than Consequence B, I ask "OK, good. If Consequence A is worth a dollar, how much is Consequence B worth?" Generally, they just give you an answer in cents without giving it a second thought.

No matter how you obtain their relative weights, the scale doesn't matter for a ratio so you can give the most severe consequence a value of 1 and give the patient's lesser consequences a proportionately smaller weight and then estimate PWB/PWC for use in the Treatment Threshold calculation as outlined above.

Here's a really helpful non-verbal technique that I often use. Let's assume that I am seeing a patient with migraine and we are deciding whether to use a daily prophylactic drug or prn abortive therapy for individual headaches. After the options have been described and discussed, I use a very simple strategy for obtaining patient input. First, I tell them that there are some patients who have incapacitating migraine lasting for days several times a week and those people jump at the chance to reduce the frequency and severity of the headaches with a daily medicine. As I tell them this, I point with my hand to my far right. But then I tell them that there are many patients who have a couple of migraines a year and the headaches respond pretty well to OTC treatments. I move my hand to the far left and say "Those patients would certainly refuse to take a daily medication just to prevent that." Finally I say, "Most patients are in between" and I start leisurely waving my hand between my far right and my far left as I ask, "So where are you?" They indicate exactly where they are with their own hand between my two extremes. Sometimes they verbalize their response as well but either way, I have their answer.

Another common example is whether to initiate anti-seizure medication after a first seizure. Let's assume that none of the factors strongly associated with seizure recurrence such as structural lesions, post-traumatic seizures, familial epilepsy or a positive mini-

ROS for prior unrecognized seizures are present. Let's also assume that there were no avoidable factors present known to be associated with provoked seizures such as severe sleep deprivation, unusual physical or psychological stress, or taking drugs such as ciprofloxacin, which would indicate a low risk of seizure recurrence.

The most useful approach is a simple discussion with the patient to show them that we are near equipoise and do not have a strong recommendation. I like to use Ben Franklin's recommendation to use self-deprecating humor to lighten the mood. That is, make fun of yourself. First I explain that we cannot predict who will have a seizure recurrence or when. "It could be years from now." Then I explain that neurologists are nearly equally divided on this point, about half would recommend treatment and half would wait for a second seizure. Then, following Franklin, I say, "When I ask people whether they would want to take a daily medication to prevent further seizures, some people say, "You want to know if I want to prevent having more seizures? Are you crazy? Of course I do." But then I tell them, "Other people say, "You want me to take medication every day to prevent a seizure and you don't even know if I'll ever have another? Are you crazy? Of course not." Then I add, "Either way, I'm crazy, so how do <u>you</u> feel about this?" It always gets a bit of a laugh, relieves the tension and gives the patient a little space to think. You get the idea.

The simplest way to involve the family is to have them present during your conversations with the patient. Sometimes this isn't possible or the patient prefers not. When appropriate, there may be separate sessions with the family. I virtually always let the patient know that I will be having family discussions so they "can ask questions." In addition to providing more information about the clinical factors already discussed, families often introduce additional factors into the decisions, including the patient's social situation, ethnic cultural values and family resources. The family can help to confirm information obtained directly from the patient. All of this information is valuable as you weave your scientific knowledge and clinical artistry into the best possible decision for your patient.

Disease Specific Factors Affecting the Benefit/Cost Ratio and Thresholds

The last chapter ended by implying that Differential Diagnosis is much more than a simple list of diagnoses ordered by statistical likelihood. In fact, there are many disease related factors, especially the natural history and how treatable, that influence our differential.

Diseases which are progressing rapidly or have the potential for producing irreversible harm with minimal warning require our immediate attention. The surgeons use an expression that I love. "What can turn around and bite you in the ass?" The idea is that before you leave the bedside you should ask yourself this question and make sure that you have considered what irreversible catastrophes could occur without warning and which could have been prevented if you had just thought about it. Sound advice!

Personally, I'd rather diagnose a treatable disorder than an untreatable disorder. I'm sure that's true for all physicians. Thus, ability to treat is a key factor altering the order of disease in your differential diagnosis. You object that we can't change what is, we have to treat the diagnosis that the patient has, not what we want it to be. True, but the question is how we proceed before we have established the diagnosis. Let's assume that after complete testing you estimate a probability of 46% for an untreatable disease and 37% for a treatable disease. Which entity is higher in your differential? More importantly, what do you do? If the patient's symptoms are evolving slowly and you judge low risk of sudden worsening, you can observe. But if the symptoms are progressing rapidly with risk of permanent loss of function, wouldn't you consider treating the less likely but disease? The answer depends on how treatable that disease is. How effective are the treatments and how severe are the potential treatment-related side effects?

This illustrates a saying of my Aunt Milly. "Go where you want to park!" That is, if you can't find a place to park your car, then where should you continue looking? Her answer was to look in the vicinity closest to your final destination. At least that way, if you do find a spot, you are where you want to be. In medicine that means that you want to help your patient improve. If you can't decide on the diagnosis but one disease is treatable and another not, it makes sense to hope that your patient has the treatable disease, explain this to the patient and recommend treatment. Go where you want to park.

Treatment can also affect testing in a negative manner when "the treatment is worse than the disease." If the patient knows in advance that they will not consent to a therapeutic procedure or if they consider the side effects of the treatment unacceptable, then there is little point in performing an invasive tests to secure that diagnosis. Unnecessary risks are never justified. Find a different course of treatment, perhaps palliative, perhaps entering a research trial, perhaps transfer to another medical center with greater clinical expertise for the patient's condition.

Remember also that one of the great advantages of Bayesian inference is that test results can be concatenated. The practical point is that sometimes it is possible to avoid an invasive test with a series of non-invasive tests, each of which lacks sufficient sensitivity and specificity to move you to the Treatment Threshold but which, together can alter the probability sufficiently that you would treat if they are all positive. Whenever you are considering an invasive test, especially if the patient has poor tolerance or is otherwise averse to it, at least ask yourself whether a series of less invasive tests can accomplish the same end. Remember my lady with temporal arteritis.

I've been using the term treatment in a naive way thus far, implying that a single modality will cure the disease. Sometimes it does, as with B12 deficiency or hypothyroidism, or a long bone fracture. But more often, the goal of treatment is mitigation of symptoms or the prevention of the more severe consequences of the disease even if the disease itself is not eliminated.

Consider this common example. The ED calls the Stroke Team to evaluate a patient with possible TIA. We're not sure; we estimate 10% probability that this was a TIA. Not very high. But the patient is hypertensive, has mildly elevated blood sugar and a family history of stroke. I believe that there is never a good reason not to engage in stroke prevention. Even though we doubt that this was a TIA, shouldn't we manage this patient's risk factors and probably start an anti-platelet agent as well? Of course, we have to give attention to the other more likely diagnoses as well. But every doctor I know would rather prevent a stroke than treat a stroke. The Benefit/Cost ratio is huge so that my Treatment Threshold for reasonable preventive measures is very low and the patient should be treated despite the low probability while the other diagnoses are being pursued.

The important principle here is that "prevention" applies not only to reducing the risk of acquiring a disease but also to reducing the risk of a disease complication. Certainly, it is absolutely essential to recommend smoking cessation to all smokers in an effort to prevent the development of COPD, lung cancer and stroke. But sophisticated surgeons, anesthesiologists and interventionalists often think about how to reduce the risk of a complication in a patient about to undergo a procedure.

Cardiology and Neurology frequently receive pre-op consults "for clearance." Junior residents often misinterpret this request. We are not being asked if it is OK to do the procedure. With rare exception, the procedure is going to proceed, may already be scheduled. Then what is the point? The point is for the consultant to review the available clinical, lab, physiology and imaging data in order to identify risks of potential complications and to provide recommendations for how to reduce those risks. These can be among the most challenging consults we do because the problem doesn't exist yet, it is only that there is a risk. Our recommendations need to be commensurate with the risk. Ideally, any additional testing and treatments need to be addressed prior to the scheduled procedure and introduce minimal additional risk. Very often, all that is needed is focused monitoring before, during and after the procedure. However, sometimes the procedure must be postponed and, very rarely, the procedure is canceled or modified to substitute a less risky procedure. You can think of it as an opportunity to reduce the Cost of treatment. I love this type of consult! It is my privilege to participate with a team providing that thoughtful level of care and I NEVER leave the consult in writing until I've discussed my understanding of the patient with the consulting team.

It is important to remember that the Cost of treating a patient includes risks that accrue during diagnosis. As already mentioned, most diagnostic procedures carry risk of harm along with the financial cost, time and potential discomfort. Also the AUC of diagnostic tests is rarely 1.0, that is, tests rarely have perfect sensitivity and specificity. This brings us to the third group of factors which alter our judgements about testing and treatment, and how we set our thresholds. This concerns the capabilities of our own medical center.

Medical Center Specific Factors Affecting the Benefit/Cost Ratio and Thresholds

One of the benefits of the decision making approach that we have developed is that the Benefit and Costs, including treatment outcomes and risks, and the sensitivity, specificity and risk of testing, all have been embedded into our decisions. I want to make one more important point, however.

Thus far we have used values for sensitivity, specificity and risk for tests from the literature. The same has been true for treatment outcomes and risks. But we do not treat patients "in the literature," we treat them in our medical center. An essential factor of our judgement in making decisions must therefore include the capabilities of our medical center.

At the extreme, your medical center may not even offer the necessary diagnostic tests, procedures or medical expertise (think ECMO or CAR T-cell therapy). If that therapy is needed then transfer to another medical center may be the only option. However, and you need to trust me on this, transfer of a patient involves its own set of risks. I have had a patient herniate and die during transfer. Transfer always involves considerable time that may increase the risk of complications if the disease is evolving rapidly. The risks of transfer obviously increase with less stable patients. These risks need to be considered in the decision to transfer; it should not be an automatic knee-jerk reaction.

You need to understand the expertise of your medical center for specific medical conditions. Very few medical centers are uniformly capable of treating all diseases or organ systems at the highest level. Some of your programs may have demonstrated outcomes that are significantly better than the literature, some may not match the results of the best centers which publish in the literature.

The same is true for diagnostic tests. You might think. "Well, an MRI is an MRI. Right?" Unfortunately, no, that is not true. Different magnets have different properties that affect the images produced. Some medical centers have older equipment or exercise less frequent tuning of the magnet to optimize imaging. The expertise and skill of the interpreting radiologists varies significantly among centers. That's also true of the pathologists who interpret biopsies. Then there are tests which are "operator dependent." That means that the technical aspects of the test take a long time to learn and the sensitivity and specificity of the test are dependent on the skill and experience of the technician. So you need to have an assessment of the skills of YOUR hospital's physicians, procedural teams and technicians. Furthermore, individual techs within your medical center may vary in their skills. I cannot emphasize this point enough. You must know the capabilities of the members of your team. Part of the art of medicine involves knowing when the literature is an accurate reflection of your medical center as well as when it might be better to wait until the right person is available or when the patient should be transferred. Your past experiences are invaluable to help form your judgements. I frequently scrub in with new surgeons and

I observe interventionalists from the control room to watch their techniques. I make mental notes of technician quality. At very least, in all cases, a face-to-face discussion prior to an invasive diagnostic procedure is essential to ensure that the person performing the invasive procedure knows exactly what information you hope to learn as well as to minimize the risks for your patient. You will be able to sense the confidence and experience of the interventionalist. Maybe the most dangerous part is not necessary and can be omitted or delayed. Maybe the patient is marginally cooperative and the key part of the test should take place at the beginning of the procedure., or involve an anesthesiologist for conscious sedation I cannot possibly overstate the importance of face to face communications prior to complex testing.

Finally, your decisions require that you take your own skills, comfort levels and availability into account. Maybe you are the only person at your medical center that performs a particular procedure and you are leaving for a rare, well-earned vacation with your family tomorrow. Maybe you are not familiar with this particular disease or medical regimen.

All of these factors alter the Benefit/Cost ratio and therefore alter the Treatment and Testing Thresholds, and have direct consequences that should be considered when you make medical decisions for your patients. The patient's outcome and safety always must come first but finding that "Best Path" is an art that will challenge you throughout your career.

How to Manage a Patient When you Have not Crossed Either Threshold

This has been a long and complex chapter. It's time to bring it to a close. The last topic is how to manage a patient in whom you have not yet crossed the treatment threshold after exhausting all available tests.

Some patients have mild non-specific symptoms, a normal exam, normal labs, physiology and imaging, and no accumulating disability despite persistent complaints. Most likely you will choose to monitor that patient clinically. See them in your clinic as follow-up. This is the most common scenario by far when you are not ready to treat. You may find that the symptoms disappear or that the underlying process declares itself over time. My mentor Dr. Dreifuss used to joke that you should maintain a long appointment wait time if you want to be known as a good diagnostician. Or maybe you will read something, learn from another patient or obtain suggestions from a colleague which tip you off as to a different direction to follow.

There are other times, however, where your patient is experiencing uncomfortable symptoms such as headaches or where your patient actually is accumulating some disability, such as from dystonia, dementia or gait disorders. Or the equivalent in other fields of medicine. Then what?

In other words, you are motivated to treat but don't have a firm diagnosis. In that case, the answer may well be to conduct a therapeutic trial. This is the firmest example of the close relationship between differential diagnosis and treatment. In this case, there is a dual purpose to your treatment, both to help the patient improve and to make the diagnosis.

Let's expand on this with one more brief example.

Example. Vestibular Migraine or Meniere's Disease
Vestibular Migraine and Meniere's Disease can produce very similar symptoms. While there are some clinical clues or audio-vestibular testing that may favor one diagnosis or the other, in certain patients it is impossible to distinguish the two diagnoses. Furthermore, the two diagnoses may co-exist in some patients. What to do?

Many physicians would resort to a therapeutic trial. This is an option when you have drugs for each condition that are relatively effective and safe within the time frame of a trial. For instance you could use acetazolamide which is an effective drug for Meniere's Disease or gabapentin which is reasonably good for migraine. Both are safe. Follow the patient's clinical response and side effects. If your first choice works, then you are done. If there was no response, then treat the second disease. If there was a response but the patient had side effects, use another drug specific for th e same disease.

This is not the only approach to a therapeutic trial, however. For one thing, a response or side effects may occur due to a placebo affect. A more time consuming approach which is less prone to placebo or bias is to conduct an n-of-1 experiment. Chose one or two drugs for each disease and then solicit the help of a colleague or pharmacist to establish a schedule alternating the drugs and including washout periods. Both you and the patient are blinded as to the drug sequence. Have the patient keep a daily diary with a simple scale of benefit and side effects that you create together. When they return to clinic at the end of the trial with their diary, you break the code and are very likely to have the answer about which drug was most effective and, often, the diagnosis along with it. I have done this numerous times in clinic when I had clinical uncertainty as to the best treatment course. It was nearly always helpful.

What if the two diseases could be treated by a single agent? For example, you could treat either generalized epilepsy or migraine with valproate. Some physicians might argue that it is more important to help the patient than to make the diagnosis. Others would argue that knowing the diagnosis is fundamental and instead would choose to use drugs which treat one diagnosis but not the other. Both approaches seem reasonable to me, it depends on the patient's clinical details and preferences, as well as the physician's practice style.

Chapter Summary

From our first simple example of *Treatment Benefit without Treatment Risk* we have traveled a long way to our final complex , real-world example of *Decisions Involving Uncertain Diagnosis, Treatment with Risks That Differ From the Disease Consequences, Using Testing With*

Risks, and Taking Patient Values into Consideration.

Wow!

The common thread throughout the chapter has been how to establish and use the Benefit/Cost ratio to select the Treatment and Testing Thresholds which guide your testing and therapeutic decisions. Focusing on a few tools, we have established a firm theoretical background and a series of practical guidelines to help organize our patient care decisions.

Medical decisions virtually always involve uncertainty. We almost never have enough information. That's where our art meets the science. It's called judgement. And don't forget to take the values of your patients into account when exerting that judgement.

Here are a few excellent references that have contributed to this chapter.

1. Therapeutic Decision Making: A Cost-Benefit Analysis. Pauker SG, Kassirer JP. NEJM 293:229-234, 1975.
2. The Threshold Approach to Clinical Decision Making. Pauker SG, Kassirer JP. NEJM 302:1109-1117, 1980.
3. THERAPEUTIC REASONING, UNC School of Medicine Christopher A. Klipstein (based on material originally prepared by Drs. Arthur Evans and John Perry)
https://www.med.unc.edu/medclerk/wp-content/uploads/sites/877/2018/10/TR5_000.pdf

Chapter 6. The "Rules" of Radiology

When I trained in Internal Medicine and then Neurology, there were no CT scans and no MRI's. Localization by the neurologic exam was almost all we had. You could get a skull X-ray, a pneumoencephalogram (I can still hear the patients cry out in pain from the air in their head), a contrast myelogram or a carotid angiogram by direct carotid stick. I remember that the first non-invasive tests were low resolution nuclear medicine brain scans and an ultrasound to see if the pineal gland was calcified and, if so, was it in the midline. You cannot imagine what a miracle our modern imaging is or how much it has changed the practice of medicine. So, no matter what area of medicine you plan to enter, you should devote yourself to learning the relevant imaging in as much detail as possible.

This very short chapter offers my advice for how clinicians should learn to use radiology to the fullest extent possible. The chapter is not about using imaging technology and certainly not about neuroimaging. There will not be any images. It is more about how to learn to use imaging and obtain the maximum benefit for your patients. There are plenty of good books and online tools to help you learn to read images. However, the best way to learn radiology is to make learning part of your patient care, just as you do for everything else. Although my focus is on clinicians who are seeing the patient, future radiologists will gain from knowing these "rules" as well.

The Five "Rules" of Radiology for Clinicians

I recommend you follow these five "Rules" of Radiology at all times. Specific comments are provided for each "Rule."

Rule #1: If you order an image, look at it!

Rule #2: Before you look at an image, know what it is going to show.

Rule #3A: If you don't know what you are looking at, find someone who does.
Rule #3B: Or read the report and figure it out.

Rule #4: Always approach imaging in a methodical manner. Do not let Rule #2 prevent you from approaching the imaging study systematically.

Rule #5: There is no substitute for a face to face conversation between clinicians and radiologists while sharing images to achieve the best patient care.

Comments on the Rules

Rule #1 is the key. When you order imaging for a patient, it means or should mean, that you have unanswered questions about your patient. You need more information. Presumably you have thought a great deal about the information you learned from the history, exam and preliminary labs. But you need more information, either because you are uncertain about the nature of the disease or need confirmation before proceeding to treat, or that you are following the progress of your patient. Those questions and the need for more information in the clinical context, set you up to learn when you review the imaging that you ordered. Does it answer your questions? How? How does it help you understand the patient's symptoms and the disease process so you are a better clinician for the next patient that you see? Does it leave more questions to be answered by other technologies? What are the limitations of the imaging modality that you used? Learning from a book or digital media is not the same because you are not "in query mode." It's valuable but not the same as learning radiology while you care for patients.

Rule #2 is meant to have you think about the imaging before you look at it. First of all, that contributes to the learning as discussed for Rule #1. But it also creates the possibility of surprise. If you don't have an expectation, you can't be surprised. Without surprise you will miss out on a lot of fun as well as the most useful learning experiences.

When your expectation is not confirmed on imaging but an alternative finding is present instead, you will be driven to read and think more about both entities, to discuss them both with your colleagues and you WILL deeply internalize your learning around both clinical entities. In general, doctors don't like surprises but surprises do usually present the best learning opportunities and they certainly add spice to our lives.

Rule #5 virtually always increases your knowledge as well as that of the radiologist, and gives rise to a higher level of thinking that improves patient care. You both learn more about the patient and the patient's disease. And be sure to document it in your progress note when you discuss the patient's imaging with a radiologist or other specialist (see also Chapter 17).

Furthermore, when you work side by side with your institution's radiologists, you will learn the reading characteristics of each radiologist with whom you work. You also will hear the level of confidence that they have in their reading in a manner that cannot be found in the official report. We have previously emphasized the importance of uncertainty in the data that you use for decision making. Given the major role that imaging plays in differential diagnosis and decisions, knowing the confidence of the radiologist in the reported findings is invaluable.

Radiologists are not technicians, they are doctors! Therefore, it is wise to discuss the patient with them as if they were a consultant BEFORE you order the image. Discuss the patient's problem with them, focusing on the information you hope to obtain from the study. They may have a better idea for how to get that information than the imaging study you were going to order. By the way, the same may be said of pathologists. They also are not technicians but rather physicians with unique experience and knowledge that can be of great value to you and your patients.

Here's an example from which you can learn at my cost. When

transesophageal ECHO (TEE) was first introduced, I ordered one for a stroke patient in order to visualize the great vessels coming off the aorta. To my surprise, when I looked at the images, I couldn't find them. I went to my favorite cardiologist and asked if I was missing the vessels or if they had not completed the study. He responded, "You can't see the great vessels with a TEE." I countered, "But that's why I ordered the test." He retorted, "I don't care, you're not going to see them with that test." End of conversation. I should have discussed it with him first.

You will encounter similar episodes from time to time. The radiologist asks why there wasn't contrast, or why there was contrast, or why an ultrasound wasn't ordered instead. So if you are certain, based on your experience, which test is the most appropriate, then go ahead and order it. But when you are facing a diagnostic challenge, it is usually best to confer with the radiologist in order to design the study together. Another benefit of this approach is that the radiologist will often offer to "protocol" the study or even directly oversee the study in order to optimize the chances of answering your question. You can't beat that!

Regarding Rule #3 A and B, it may be more efficient to follow Rule #3B but you certainly will not learn as much as following Rule #3A.

Finally, regarding Rule #4, there is a story that is told about Dr. Lucy Squire, radiologist and educator at Downstate Medical Center from 1966 to 1994, and author of the wildly popular book *Fundamentals of Radiology*. You should read the first several chapters of that book if you have not done so already. The story about Dr. Squire goes that she always carried a chest x-ray in her coat pocket (a film, of course, this is pre-digital era) and she would periodically put the film up for students to read. She said that she could always tell which students would make good radiologists because "they were the last one to see the tumor in the lung, but the only one to see the metastasis in the humerus."

Get it? She is telling you to review images systematically! Your clinical bias (Rule #2) can be very useful but it must not prevent you from following Rule #4.

Modern imaging is beautiful and invaluable to advanced patient care. Be sure to learn everything that you can at every opportunity, and especially in relationship to your own patients. There is no better way to learn radiology than to correlate your clinical observations with the findings on imaging, and that will make you a better clinician as well.

Chapter 7. Working with Other Physicians, Nurses and Staff

As the saying goes, "It takes a Village." In this chapter, I will offer suggestions for how to optimize your interactions with other health care professionals. As always, the suggestions are based on personal experience, both successes and failures. Caring for patients in the modern medical era is incredibly complex. Building and embedding yourself into a team, or series of teams, is the key to your success as a physician.

The AAMC Pre-professional competencies explicitly include Teamwork. What does "Teamwork" mean in medicine? At Einstein Medical Center, every neurology residency candidate has experienced the same patterned admission interviews. One of the questions was "I would like to discuss with you the relationship between teamwork and leadership. How do you think about that?" And a discussion followed. Teamwork is a fundamental principle of our department's faculty, residency and staff. The Leader is simply a member of the team with a particular function. Like every other member, the Leader has tasks to do and responsibilities to uphold.

As a physician, you will have to assume a variety of leadership roles throughout your career because of your knowledge, skills, experience and decision making responsibilities. Whether caring for a particular patient, improving your hospital unit or clinic, organizing a task force to improve on a new or a problematic function, helping your medical center provide optimal care for your community, conducting medical research or helping define national or international standards and goals, you will be part of teams. Learning when and how to lead and when and how to participate without leading are important skills for every physician. The healthcare system depends on our ability to perform both roles.

Personally, I have found a few principles to be consistently useful guides. Some of these may seem small and insignificant. In some ways they are, but leadership is not always about the big role. Sometimes very small actions can have very big consequences, either in a positive or negative way.

First, second, third and fourth is to remember that our purpose is to care for patients. Any time the best course is unclear, ask yourself what would be best for the patient. Also, I have said hundreds of times "Never fix the system while taking care of a patient." That is bad for the patient, bad for you and bad for the system. Don't do it! Take care of the patient. Then fix the system.

A patient who had observed me following this rule said to me, "What I like about you is that you don't have a big ego that gets in the way." I laughed and said, "Oh, no. You have it all wrong. My ego is so big that those things don't matter to me." She laughed. I don't know if she was right or I was right but, either way, the point is that you should never let egos interfere with patient care. Unfortunately, they can and do. The result is almost always regrettable. Throughout your career you will find that you need to take an action that you know is someone else's responsibility. Which service admits the patient? Who does the discharge summary? Who should take the stat blood work to the lab? You'll see, it will happen. If a quick discussion doesn't correct the problem, then take care of the patient and sort out the issue later.

Another important principle is to treat everyone on your healthcare team with respect and understanding. Ideally, know them by name. When I work in the ED with a nurse that I haven't met, I immediately ask the nurse's name and introduce myself. From that moment, we are a team caring for the patient on the stretcher. Also, I am always eager to help in any little way that I can, to save the nurse a trip around the stretcher by adjusting the IV or handing the patient the urinal. And I thank the nurse when we are done and let them know what a great job they did and what a pleasure it was working with them and how I look forward to working with them again. Each joint episode of patient care builds upon the last. Soon the nurse and I are a strong and efficient team capable of anticipating each other's needs. We actually look forward to working together again. And when the unexpected complication arises suddenly, we are capable of addressing it efficiently and effectively. Maybe we even anticipated the possibility and were already preparing or had acted to prevent it.

We will discuss compassion for patients in a later chapter but there also is a role for compassion when you interact with team members. All of us who experienced the full force of the COVID-19 pandemic or other large scale disasters are aware of how exhausting a prolonged, full and continuous effort can be. Supplies are not the only thing that run short. So do patience, tolerance and empathy. A good team knows how to recognize and give extra help when a member is affected by injury or unusual stress.

Buddha says, "We reap in times of need what we sow in times of plenty." In other words, it is easiest to build a team while stress is low. The cohesion of the team is a major factor that allows it to overcome the unexpected stresses that inevitably arise. Building a team is a continuous process. You are always doing it, it never stops. How? By knowing names, saying "Good Morning," looking people in the eye, treating them with respect, being ready to lend a hand, learning from each other at every opportunity and engaging in group thought. Mutual respect, support and responsibility are the keys to the success of a healthcare team.

And we never point a finger when a "mistake" occurs. Anyway, most mistakes are indications that the system didn't work correctly. Mistakes and "near misses" are opportunities to improve the system, without blame. I also believe that "In order for there to be a screw-up, EVERYONE has to screw up. Because if even ONE person doesn't screw up, then there is no screw-up." We are all responsible for the actions of our team. Redundancy of independent thinking is a major prophylactic against screw-ups.

By the way, my pronouns are "We, Us and Our." When the Northport VAMC was preparing for its Joint Commission Survey, our motto was: There is no "They" there is only "We."

Emergencies and Urgent Situations

In soccer, there is a riddle that goes, "Who is the team leader?" The answer is, "The player closest to the ball." Everyone must be ready to lead at the appropriate moment. This is particularly relevant during patient care emergencies. The person in charge must be clear to everyone involved. If I am joining a Code Blue, Stroke Alert or Rapid Response in progress, I immediately ask, "Who's in charge here?" And I direct my questions and thoughts directly to them. If you are in charge, you need to speak and act in a manner that makes that clear to the rest of the team so they know to whom they should provide their input and to make sure that you are aware of all actions being taken. Failure to do so leads to disorganized care.

It is also important to keep in mind that staff availability varies during time of day. Many more people will show up in an emergency during the daytime than in the middle of the night. In some ways, as long as the right people are present, the smaller team can be an advantage but it requires a more thoughtful approach to delegation of responsibilities. Staff availability and responsibilities at night or weekends may also dictate a change in venue for the patient to a unit staffed for a higher level of care.

I have found that the best teams have a discussion after the emergency passes, whether successful or not. The leader should give and receive feedback with the rest of the team. What went well, what did not, what were the crucial junctures, what might have been done differently? And, assuming that the patient survives, it is extremely valuable to obtain follow-up the next day or two to understand what happened and how the patient has faired. A good team, a good medical center, facilitates this type of feedback naturally.

Let's move on to some specific relationships.

Consultants

Most doctors will stand on both sides of this line. We both are and use consultants. Consultants are your colleagues. They are doctors, physician extenders or therapists that you ask for advice and assistance, sometimes one and sometimes both, and *vice versa*. Here are my bits of advice for being admired as a consultant and getting the most out of your consultants.

Let's begin by focusing on the relationship between referring practitioner and consultant. The referring doctor is taking care of a patient and believes that further assistance of a doctor from another field would be helpful. Why? There are many possible answers. The referrer:

- may not yet be comfortable with the differential diagnosis, or
- is comfortable with the differential diagnosis but needs a specialist for a diagnostic test, or
- knows the diagnosis but wants the help of a specialist for administration of a complex medical regimen, or
- believes that the patient may need a procedure as part of treatment, or
- believes that another type of practitioner would be better able to provide long-term care, or
- simply wants to re-assure the family that the patient's current management has been optimized, or
- many other reasons.

Here are some principles of consultations.

The consultant has the right to expect that the referrer has

1. clearly expressed a specific question, even if it is for help with diagnosis,
2. indicated whether there is urgency involved,
3. notified the patient that a consultation with another doctor has been requested and why, and
4. made a good effort to ensure that all available information is readily available for the consultant.

The referrer has the right to expect that the consultant will

1. thoroughly evaluate the patient with an independently performed history and physical exam,
2. review available pertinent labs, electrophysiology and imaging,
3. formulate a differential diagnosis independently of the referrer,
4. communicate back with a clear diagnostic impression and management recommendations, including any further diagnostic tests, treatments or further consultations, along with a sense of urgency.

Let me share my experience as a consultant at Fox Chase Cancer Center. Einstein is close to Fox Chase and our faculty welcomed the opportunity to do consultations on their very complex patients. Their use of consultations was incredible and can serve as an example for all of us. We would be notified of a pending consult by a secretary by phone with a very brief history and a specific question. The expectation was that the patient would be seen within 24 hours, if more urgent, the physician called instead and asked to speak with our department's consultant for that day. Upon arrival on the patient's unit, a nurse would greet us, ask if we needed coffee, hand us the paper chart, offer to open the electronic record for us and show us where the patient's room was. If the patient was not in their room, they would find the patient for us and together we would decide where the consultation should occur. Before we entered the room, the referring Attending appeared, thanked us for coming, explained the patient's past care, reiterated and discussed the reason for the referral and asked if anything else was needed. After the consult, upon leaving the patient's room, the Attending would appear either immediately or, certainly, before I could get very far in writing the note. We would discuss my findings and opinions, maybe review imaging and labs together, possibly speak with an earlier consultant, and then formulate a plan jointly. That is about as perfect as perfect can be. It should be a model for all of us. It is the model we strive for on our Neuroscience Unit at Einstein.

Certain issues between referrer and consultant are not as uniformly agreed upon and may vary from patient to patient. Most importantly, how much should the consultant share with the patient before speaking with the referring doctor? That varies a great deal by referrer, less so by patient. I will reiterate that the patient must know in advance that another doctor will be coming to see them as a consultant. I also believe, that the consultant should be aware of the referrer's expectation for how much information the consultant will share with the patient before speaking to the referring doctor. Since I try to have a conversation with the referrer before seeing the patient, I ask specifically what they would like me to discuss with the patient and family. If I'm not sure, my usual practice is to tell the patient and family, after the history and physical, that I want to review the labs, electrophysiology and imaging again, "now that I know them better." While I'm doing that or organizing my note, I call the referring doctor (or team), let them know my thoughts and then ask them what I can share with the patient. Why do that?

Because "mixed messages" are very disturbing to the patient and family and should be avoided at all cost. If I have a different opinion than the referrer, I will share that with the patient, of course, but, by having a conversation with the referrer first, I have a better understanding of why the referrer held the original position. That allows me to formulate a cohesive explanation to the patient that helps them understand our areas of uncertainty and gives them confidence that we have worked and will continue to work together to resolve those issues.

Patient satisfaction is important for many reasons. Once I wanted to better understand our Neuroscience Unit's satisfaction scores. As usual, I simply asked the patients and families directly myself. My two part question was, "Would you give us a 9 or 10?" Whether they answered yes or no, my follow-up question was, "Why?" I interviewed 10 families. We got a yes 8 times and no twice. But, amazingly, ALL 10 FAMILIES gave the SAME answer for "Why?" Their answer was strictly related to whether they perceived that the whole team was communicating with one another. If they thought we were, we got 9 or 10. If not, we didn't. "But what about the rooms, the food, the noise?" "Well, yeah, but this isn't a hotel. We're here for medical care." Perception of communication among all team members was the ONLY answer I received from the patients and families. Make it happen!

There is one issue about referrers and consultants that drives me nuts. Once the consultant leaves recommendations, is the referrer bound to follow all of them? NO! A consultant is a consultant and that's all. Sure, the consultant may know more about some specific topic but the referrer probably knows more about this specific patient and family, including their values and preferences. A good consultant will be aware of some but not necessarily all. As a consultant, I accept that the referrer has the final say and may accept or reject my recommendations. When I am the referrer, I assure you that I do not feel compelled to slavishly follow the recommendations of my consultants. However, if decide not to follow a recommendation, I will discuss it with the consultant to make sure I understand their view of the patient. They might change my mind.

That's why conversations are so important. Ideally, the consultant has the good sense to express their charted recommendations in terms that are less than adamant. "Consider MRI for possible spine tumor" or "Patient may achieve better BP control if . . ." When the consultant feels strongly about a recommendation, it is their <u>responsibility</u> to make that strong feeling known to the referrer along with why. It is also expected that the referrer will explicitly address in their progress notes why they are not following a strong recommendation of the consultant if they don't. We'll discuss notes again later.

Sometimes therapists are the consultants. That can create some interesting situations, especially for stroke patients. Therapists are strong patient advocates. Let's assume that they recommend inpatient rehab but the patient's insurance won't cover that, or that the patient or family refuses. As the attending, how shall I react? Well, first of all, the therapist and I will already have discussed this issue at Discharge Planning Rounds (see below). So we would try to formulate an alternative plan, maybe relying more on the family. The therapist and I often go to the bedside to examine the patient together for safety concerns. We agree on limits to care that are necessary for patient safety and then work together to find the best alternative. Every case resolves differently. The process, however, always involves joint problem solving. Ultimately, as the referring Attending, I'm responsible for the patient. I believe that there can be only one captain of a ship. The Attending of record, whether inpatient or outpatient, has the final say. I respect that rule, whichever side of the consultation that I am on.

One last point on this important relationship has to do with the value of providing follow-up information between referrer and consultant. Frequently, the patient's care is continued by one of the physicians but not both. When that happens, it is a huge bonus for the one providing ongoing care to share outcome or progress with the other when they happen to meet again (not just through notes transmitted by the EMR). "Remember Jones who had . . ., well we found . . ., and treated him with . . ., and he is doing great!" Or, "You won't believe what we found out about Jones. He . . ." The discussion that follows is a great way for both to learn as they share related experiences. Their relationship is bonded in a manner that can only be bested by joint care at the bedside. They will both look forward to the next opportunity for working together. Their patients will receive better care. So take the time to provide follow-up information about patients that you have shared. It's always appreciated and always worth while.

The Primary Care Provider (PCP)

Primary care providers, whether physician, physician's assistant or nurse practitioner, are very special referrers. They have longitudinal, multi-dimensional knowledge about the patient that virtually no one else has. But they also work with time constraints that would drive most of us nuts and they are the only providers who take care of patients with every conceivable medical problem. Their demands and constraints are unimaginable to me. I have two family doctors in my immediate family and I still don't see how they do it.

So I believe that consultants carry a special responsibility when the referrer is a PCP. We have to be the one to reach out and initiate the discussion after the consultation. In other words, pick up the phone and call them! There are many, many reasons to do this. First, they will appreciate it and have increased respect for you as well as your medical center. It is sad that they are often surprised when I call and tell them I would like to discuss their patient. There are many times that I gain additional information from the referrer after providing my opinions. "No, we tried that and it didn't work." I also feel that it is a mistake for a consultant to start a new long-term medication without discussing it first with the provider. My relationship with the patient lasts an hour or so. Theirs is life-long. Unless that was the explicit reason for the consult, why should my medication preference force the physician to continue a drug for years? They might have their own drug preferences once they know the condition. They might already have tried it and the patient didn't respond. There may be additional factors which, unknown to me, might add risks to the treatment I am considering. "The patient has had depression . . ." or "The patient was addicted to . . ." In general, I talk fast and keep the conversation to the point, they have huge workloads. But, if I detect a more relaxed attitude, then its nice to be able to slow down and chat. And strengthen a relationship!

I always ask the patient who their PCP is. When they tell me, I let them know how well I know the person. If possible, if I have had experience with the PCP, I let the patient know. "Oh, yea. We've worked together before." Or, "Oh, sure, I know her very well, we've worked together a lot." And unless you absolutely don't agree with this statement, add "Your lucky, she's really good." And finally, "We'll make sure to share everything that we learn with her." Doing that eliminates a whole host of patient concerns. Of course that means a conversation and letter with discharge summary to the PCP.

My sister-in-law, Dr. Alida Evans, is a family physician. She would like to add that the family doctor's continuity of care enriches their appreciation of each patient's values. This mutual knowledge is often instrumental when patients are under duress such after a stroke or being diagnosed with cancer. She reinforces my own comments above by adding that "this knowledge is rarely tapped by hospitalists." Historically, PCP's used to do their patient's hospital admissions and coordinate ongoing hospital care. This ensured incorporation of patient and family values, as well as the patient's prior decision-making. This knowledge can be invaluable in Goals of Care discussions.

As an example, in the 1990's, I was caring for a 94 year old woman in the ED with a potentially significant acute stroke. The ED doctor was reluctant to give tPA outside of the current recommendations but the patient had been independent and I favored thrombolysis. We agreed to call her PCP and let the PCP provide input. When I asked the PCP if we should give tPA, she shouted "You'd better! She's our Fourth in bridge! We did and the patient recovered fully, including playing bridge.

At the Northport VA we believed that "A patient care team without a PCP is like a wheel without a hub. It just won't roll."

Nurses

The relationship between doctor and nurse is special and unique, there is probably no other like it in any other human undertaking. In my opinion, it is at the center of healthcare. The bond that grows through the shared experiences of patient care evades description. The beauty of the relationship is that for all of the commonality of goals and scientific knowledge, our relation to the patient differs fundamentally in important ways, especially in the hospital. We'll talk about doctor - patient relationships later but the nurse is nearly always closer to the patient than the doctor in the ED or hospital, and now a days even in the clinic. Sure, the doctor is hands on for exam and a good doctor might help the nurse get the patient undressed and other things. I've been known to clean the glasses of a patient with dirty lenses. But the nurse is ALWAYS hands on. A good nurse uses their closeness to obtain information from the patient that the patient might not share initially with the doctor. The nurse simply spends more time with them, certainly that is true in the hospital and ED.

Nurses also tend to be more aware of the family and social interactions of the patient outside of the hospital, including financial, interpersonal problems and complex relationships in the home. These can be of crucial importance for successfully planning ongoing patient care. It is important to find an opportunity to learn about these factors from the patient's nurse.

There is simply something that I cannot describe about addressing an emergency with a good, confident nurse. Your roles differ but there is no dividing line and the overlap is enormous and fluid. And when the patient is stabilized and you can both slow down and reflect, there's a glow between you. And I cannot emphasize the next point enough. Say "Thank you, you did a great job!" But then also let them know what the monitoring VS and exam parameters are going forward, along with frequency, and exactly what your plan is along with your expectation for when elements of the plan are completed. And give them your cell phone so they can contact you immediately and directly, without using a paging system, in case there are unexpected clinical events or the plan cannot be executed in a timely manner. This is respectful, it is friendly and it re-enforces the importance that you place on tight monitoring going forward. These are not mutually exclusive features.

The attendings and residents who spend time in the Einstein Neuroscience Unit (NSU) all share a very close working relationship with our nurses. Our attitude toward our unit nurses is built upon the belief that hospital medicine is too complicated for any one person; that consistently positive patient outcomes only come from redundancy. That is, the faculty depends on multiple levels of independent thinkers working with them. It is our expectation that our residents, our students, our nurses, therapists and clerks all are looking at the patient with a clinical eye independently and making sure that things are going well, letting us know if not.

We also involve our housekeeping, transportation and food personnel, We reinforce this for this latter group through regular discussions, education and expressions of gratitude. We involve them in our parties and our Joint Commission surveys as part of the team. You may have heard that during preparation for our first flight to the moon, a housekeeper at NASA was asked what his role was there. His response was "I'm helping to land someone on the moon." And so he was.

Back to our nurses. I always remind them that "With responsibility, comes responsibility." These are their patients as much as mine. They should not administer a drug if they do not understand why I ordered that drug. They should not transport the patient for a test if our team hasn't discussed the test with them beforehand. I expect them to demand that, I demand that they demand it. If a patient is called for a test that we have not discussed, they should call me or our team before transporting the patient. If a physician not on the Neurology inpatient team orders a medication, they should let us know before they give that med. They should feel free to ask the doctor if they had discussed the specific drug and dosage with the Neurology team. And if the plan that we prescribed is not having the expected effect, they should let us know immediately. They can call a Rapid Response, they can initiate a Stroke Code. Our nurses receive the same clinical education as our residents along with their nursing specific education. They can ask us anything they want any time they want. Some of our nurses have been on our unit for more than a decade. They know what they are doing and we trust them. Our respect and support are mutual. Of course we also celebrate together on holidays and birthdays, as well as any other excuse we can find.

And I hug. When a nurse saves a patient's life or averts a catastrophe through their quick and thoughtful action, I don't know any other way to thank them enough.

Other Staff

This is a ridiculously large category that includes the clerical staff, therapists, lab and technical staff, aides, medical assistants, housekeeping, transport, pharmacy and administration that contribute to the success of every inpatient or outpatient unit. You can include EMS personnel if you are in the ED.

"It takes a village." Each role listed above, and others that I might be neglecting, is essential to patient care. Remove any role and workflow comes to a stop. That brings to mind that "A chain is only as strong as its weakest link."

If you want to be successful as a physician, and I assume you do, then you need to create good working relationships with everyone. We are all working together, we all want what is best for our patients. We all have our own lives, with dreams and troubles. We all want to develop the best skills possible and learn as much about medicine as we possibly can. We are all interested in the behavior of patients with diseases.

So be nice! Make sure that everyone understands what you are doing with the patient. Share what you know with them. Learn from them. Some simple examples to demonstrate. Who is the best person to teach you how to adjust the appearance of an image on a screen to review imaging? Ans: A radiology tech. To evaluate a patient's rehab potential? A therapist. To put in a Foley? An ED tech. To draw blood? A phlebotomist. To complete a request form? A clerk. Get it? All of these people have learned skills that can be useful to you. You teach them, they teach you. We are all in this together. We all want to enjoy our jobs.

As far as I'm concerned, stress is pretty useless and interferes with smooth patient care. It's damn unpleasant. There's already enough stress just taking care of patients, medicine is hard. We should always strive to minimize the stress in our lives and work.

If I encounter someone who seems not to have the patient's best interest in mind, who doesn't want to learn, who regularly increases stress or is otherwise unpleasant as a colleague, I immediately bring it to their supervisor's attention. A bad apple spoils the bunch. If one person is allowed to behave that way, then it invariably reduces the satisfaction of everyone else on the team and increases the risk that other's behave badly.

Conversely, when I encounter someone who consistently goes above and beyond, whether in terms of learning, responsibility, skill levels, initiative, patient relations, I do several things. First, I let that person know that I am impressed. Second, if appropriate, I ask them what their career goals are. Third, I ask if there is anything I can do to help them achieve those goals. Can I write a letter for them, open a door, make a recommendation? Fourth, I let their supervisor know that they have a person with strong potential on their team. Often they already know, but they are always glad to hear some kind words. And, you gain respect for noticing and for caring enough to take the time to do something about it. "It takes one to know one."

Discharge Planning Rounds

From the first day of our Stroke Unit at Stony Brook in 1996, through my time at Wisconsin and until my last day of work at Einstein in 2024, I participated every day that I was on service in Discharge Planning Rounds. "It is 15 minutes that will save you 2 hours every day." It also is a key factor in building your team. If anything can help with length of stay, this is it.

Everyone on the unit involved in patient care comes or is represented if too busy with immediate care. Every patient on the unit is discussed. History, exam, differential, tests and consults for the day, issues related to family, drugs, therapies, procedures and, of course, discharge issues are all discussed for every patient. That includes issues related to insurance. And, on average, each patient gets about one minute. Nuts? No, you just have to focus and avoid unnecessary info. There's almost always time for a little teaching and always time to discuss complex patient issues. At the end, I like to finish with a quote from Buddha. I have a copy of "Buddha's Little Instruction Book" in my white coat inside pocket from which I have read at every discharge planning rounds since 1996. Usually at random but sometimes a purposely selected saying. Buddha reminds us of our humanity. There are plenty of other options for daily inspiration of course.

As the meeting ends, it is a team that is dispersing, ready for the day.

Chapter 8. The Doctor-Patient Relationship

Learn Something From Every Patient You See.
This simple saying has stood out as the most important guideline of my career. I vaguely remember being told this by some wise clinician when I was starting medical school. I can promise you, without any reservations, that if you follow this guideline you will be an outstanding doctor.

Some patients have many things to teach, but every patient has something. You may learn something about how people report their history, or a new way of eliciting a physical finding, or a new way of interpreting a lab, or recognizing a condition on imaging, or how a particular drug interacts with other drugs, or when a surgical approach is more beneficial. But you may also learn about the importance of addressing hopelessness in your patients, or how the loss of a child can disrupt a marriage, or how certain psychologically based therapies can help patients overcome addiction.

Like every other skill that you will learn, regular, consistent use is the best strategy. Simply this, after finishing with the patient, practice asking yourself, 'What did I learn from this patient?' That's all there is to it! After 10's of thousands of patients, you will be amazed what you have learned from your patients.

The Authoritarian Approach Went Out of Style a Long Time Ago.
When I was a medical student, most doctors practiced, and were expected to practice, with an authoritarian style. Some were more benevolent than others but most believed that doctors knew the best thing for their patients and patients expected to be told what to do next.

To some extent, that is still true. When Einstein did some research about what our patients wanted, the research firm informed us that we were in trouble. Our patients wanted two things. First, they wanted to be in control of their own decision making. Second, they wanted to be told what to do. Hmmm.

Well, that dilemma aside, I am "a child of the 60's," meaning I believe in questioning authority. I never wanted an asymmetric relationship with my patients. Yes, I am the doctor with much more knowledge about their condition than they have, but they know themselves and their own value sets and their own ways of understanding.

I have often summarized my feeling to students and residents by saying simply that tomorrow, you may need your patient to fix your car.

We are both people. I have a job to do. They have come to me for help. My goal is to determine the best available options and then to educate them so that they can evaluate my recommendations. In the end, however, they may choose to follow my preferred recommendation, or a reasonable alternative or to seek another opinion. All are valid options.

I also believe, by the way, that I am not obligated to offer an option that I believe to be futile or even harmful. Fortunately, in over 44 years in practice, I have never had to refuse any treatment request on moral grounds. That is a very "slippery slope." While euthanasia is a subject that neurologists may be asked to consider, I never was. We always seemed to find a way to achieve an acceptable level of comfort care. I don't know how I would have responded if I were approached by a patient in a state where euthanasia was legal.

Professionalism

Physicians implicitly and explicitly accept a strong code of responsibility to our patients. It is understood that we will practice to the best of our ability in a compassionate manner. The problem is that the world can intrude on that commitment. We experience personal traumas, including disappointments. It is natural for us to lose confidence after an untoward result. We have fights with family members, we have financial problems, we become angry with colleagues, with our hospital administration or frustrated with medicine in general. Just like anyone else.

"Professionalism" is a term that I use for myself, as well as others, in an effort to minimize the impact of all of these extraneous factors and every other influence which is not directly related to the care of the patient in front of me. Our commitment as doctors to professionalism means that we focus on the person in front of us and give them our complete attention, attempting to satisfy their needs in the best manner available to us.

Professionalism, to me, also indicates that I must treat each person with respect, without regard to any distinguishing factor such as gender, race, beliefs or prior self-abusive behaviors. That boundary becomes very nebulous if a person engages in activities that produce harm to others, however, especially children. Such a topic is beyond the scope of this book, however.

Kadosh

The Hebrew word, Kadosh, is often interpreted as "holy" but it literally means "set aside." In Judaism, it is common to say a prayer before using something considered Kadosh such as lighting the Sabbath candles or starting a meal. Early on in my career I found it helpful to "set aside" my time with patients by pausing before entering clinic to meditate or pray in order to center myself in my role of healer and to ensure that I was focused on my patients to the exclusion of all of the other influences of my life. I still talk to myself as I am hurrying to the ED or before entering the ICU to ensure that I am fully focused on the task at hand.

Bedside Manners

I remember a much more senior faculty member making the seemingly outrageous statement at a Curriculum Committee meeting at Stony Brook that "it doesn't matter to me if a doctor cares about his patients or not." You can imagine the furious responses that this elicited. However, at the end of the hour, his point had been made that whether the doctor cared or not was less important than his or her ability to act as if they cared. Who is more effective at the bedside, the doctor who cares but can't show it or the doctor who doesn't care but conveys to the patient the feeling that he does? The goal, of course, is to achieve both. But from that raucous discussion I learned that I must act at the bedside, in the sense of being an actor, for the good of my patients.

Once that concept is accepted, however, a whole new world opens up. I mean, if your going to act at all, you might as well do it well, and with a purpose! What's the purpose? Over the years, my understanding of the purpose developed into the idea that I should become the doctor that this patient needs me to be in order to get well.

That must strike you as a bit strange so let's dwell on it a little. There are actually two tasks here. The first task is creating your "persona" for the patient and the second task is accomplishing the purpose of this particular encounter with this patient.

When we are discussing this on the ward, I usually stroke my beard obviously and say "You think that this gray is a huge advantage for me, don't you?" Everyone's eyes open wide and they nod Yes emphatically. My response to that is, "Well it is. But I was once young and naive, and that was a huge advantage to me too." In other words, we all have an advantage, we just have to realize what it is and use it to our advantage. An obvious example at Einstein had to do with the fact that 78% of our patients are African-American. When we had a black student or resident on our team, you could see, I mean physically see, the patients and families swell with pride at that trainee's involvement on our team. Even physical handicaps can be an advantage. You will have to figure out your own advantages for yourself.

As for the task at hand, it varies a great deal. Sometimes a sympathetic approach is needed, sometimes a very matter of fact approach, occasionally a somewhat harsh approach is needed such as with someone who presented with a smoking related stroke but who refuses to give up cigarettes.

How do you know who to be and how to act in the moment? Like everything else in medicine, you learn by observing more experienced physicians and from your own experience as you take care of patients, trying things out and learning what works well for you and which patient cues predict the approach that will best help achieve the patient's specific needs.

"When in Rome, do as the Romans do!" Great saying, but the problem is, what do you do when you first get to Rome? The best is to be alert and observe. Again, the more you do it, the better you get. We've already considered this problem when beginning the patient's history. We'll return to it again later.

Here's one great guideline. Dr. Chris Bradley was a super neurologist in our department, trained in epilepsy at Yale but also a fantastic generalist. I was trying to help a young faculty member whose patient satisfaction ratings were not very good. I told one of our front office clerks that I was going to interview his patients and try to find out why they weren't giving him high scores. Our clerk looked at me and said, "Wouldn't it be more useful to interview the patients of Dr. Bradley and find out why they like him so much?" Duuuh. So that's what I did. Amazingly, 10 out of 10 of his patients gave me exactly the same answer. Exactly the same! Every one of them said, "Oh, he just makes me feel so comfortable." Now you need to know that Dr. Bradley was also the busiest member of our faculty, he could see nearly twice as many patients in a session as the rest of us. So it wasn't the time he spent, it was how he spent his time. On reflection, Chris always seemed relaxed, he always wore a smile, he always seemed interested in what people had to say and when he spoke it was plain sense, spoken directly and without artifice. He could also let you know when he disagreed with something without rancor. So there's at least one successful strategy you might try. Strive to make your patients "comfortable."

Let's take up several specific topics. As always, these are my opinions based on my experience and my observations of hundreds of students, residents and faculty. Others may feel very differently on any or all of these points. You have to decide for yourself.

First Names

I recommend avoiding first names. From beginning of medical school to my retirement, I called only one patient by her first name. I am not comfortable being called by my first name, I want the patient to respect my professional position. I may need to ask them to do things that they really don't want to do. I may need to give them very bad news. I may need to point out behaviors that are contrary to their own well-being. I'm not their friend, I'm their doctor, hopefully able to show compassion. But, if they don't use my first name, then symmetry says that I don't call them by their first name. And there it is.

I introduce residents as "Doctor Jones." I introduce students as "Student Doctor Jones." After that first time, I drop the student and it's simply "Doctor Jones." Get used to it. Learn to wear it, you've earned it. In most cases, it leads to a better patient relationship. It also avoids potential pitfalls such as transference and other inappropriate behaviors. A little distance is useful in most doctor - patient relationships. And, by the way, I never once heard a patient refer to Dr. Bradley as "Chris."

No Buttons and No Scents!

No scents is obvious, patients can be allergic or have reactive airway disease. Perfumes, colognes, perfumed soaps and detergents are all out of the question. Why no buttons? In the US right now, the odds of someone agreeing with the slogan is 50-50. Right? Half of the people are going to disagree. Do you really want to begin your relationship with a 50% chance that your patient finds your outspoken stance annoying? Probably not. So, no buttons. Let's avoid unnecessary distractions and stay focused on building a good relationship and accomplishing the task at hand.

If You Don't Know, Say "I Don't Know"

I cannot emphasize how important this is. It is not at all uncommon, even after a thorough history and physical exam, that the diagnosis and ultimate management are not clear. Get used to that. The probability of that happening becomes smaller over the years but I promise you that it never goes away. You need to be able to convey this to the patient in a manner that isn't disturbing to them. Typically, I will say something like, "Well, you've been very clear about your symptoms and the exam has been helpful, but it still isn't clear exactly what is causing your symptoms." Before they have a chance to panic, you can either follow Ben Franklin's advice and use "self-deprecating humor" such as "Don't worry, that's not rare for me, so I've gotten pretty good at handling this" or you can be more straight-forward and say, "Don't get me wrong, it's not like I have no idea (hands making quotes), it's just that there are still several possibilities that might explain the problem and we're going to have to work this through." The two approaches work together as well. Continue, "So we're going to need to get a bit more information. I'm going to recommend ...." Generally, that will do the trick very nicely.

Projecting Confidence

While we're at it, lets talk about patient confidence which is not necessarily the same as satisfaction. Understandably, patients need to believe that you know what you are doing or will have the sense to seek help in an organized and useful way when you don't. Part of your acting, in the sense discussed above, needs to include this. Your demeanor needs to be calm and steady. That's particularly true in an emergency. I often find myself leaning on the bedrail or wall even as I'm leading our team at breakneck speed because I want everyone on the team to have the same confidence in our abilities that I would want the patient to have. Learning to portray an image of being relaxed and in control is invaluable to your success as a physician. The confidence will come with time. I love the line from the movie *Patton,* when after one of Patton's tirades, his adjutant says, "Sometimes they can't tell when you're serious or not," and Patton responds, "It isn't important for them to know, its only important for me to know."

Being confident in no way means that you can't ask for help or share decision making. "Any suggestions?" is a fair question to ask aloud when things are not going well. "What are we missing?" to the group is useful whether things are going well or not. I ask both regularly. Either can elicit very useful suggestions from other team members.

Transparency with the Patient

One of the most distinct evolutions in my practice during my career has been a strong and consistent tendency to become more transparent with the patient. I don't mean just being honest at all times. That's necessary and obvious but just the starting point. I mean letting them know exactly what I am doing and anticipating questions that they may have. It begins during the history. "I'm wondering whether your symptoms may be due to seizures, so the next questions are going to be about seizures." On exam, "I need to see how strong you are so, please, give me your full effort. If it hurts, just stop and say so, but otherwise I assume that you're giving me everything you've got."

We're going to deal with how to deliver bad news in detail later on so here I would just limit things to say something like, "Your exam is very consistent with the symptoms you describe. They both are pointing to a particular part of the brain [indicating on their head where] and so I think we should get a CAT scan to see if there is something there that can explain it." Then just continue, don't wait for the obvious question. "There are a lot of things that can behave this way, so instead of discussing all of them, let's just go ahead and get the test. I'll look at it and come speak with you very soon after its done."

Whether in clinic or in the ED or hospital, its usually helpful to the patient to get a sense of the time course of the workup. "Your symptoms have been present for several years and aren't progressing very quickly, so I think we can take our time working this out. That'll let us go step by step and we can avoid unnecessary tests that way." Or, "Obviously this has been moving along fairly rapidly, so I think we should not waste time but figure this out sooner rather than later in order to begin the right treatment as soon as possible. I think it would be best if you stayed in the hospital. I'm hoping to arrange an MRI for tonight or tomorrow."

Explaining treatment courses is a world of its own and I will not address that in this book because it is so diverse.

Lot´s of people have contributed a lot to this book. My sister-in-law, Dr. Evans, also wants me to emphasize how important it is to listen to what the patient has to say. She doesn´t mean just hearing the information that the patient is providing as we have emphasized thus far. Alida means to hear what the patient is telling you about themselves, or their family, and how they are reacting to the illness. What are your patient's concerns? How can you help with those?

That reminds me of a lesson that I learned as an intern. I had a patient with rapidly advanced and untreatable cancer (in 1977). I remember him say, "Just don't tell my wife, it'll kill her." Later, I was speaking to her about his condition, without using the word cancer per his request, when she said, "I know he is dying of cancer but whatever you do, don't tell him, it will break his heart." How sad! At the very moment that they should be as close as possible, his disease is creating a barrier between them. How to address this? Remember, I'm an intern at the time. Are they using this barrier as a defense mechanism that allows them to spend their last time together in peace or is it a barrier? I didn't know them anywhere near well enough to say. I opted for an approach that I would still use today. I told each of them, "Well, I think they already know and has told me so. Maybe it would be best to put that aside so you can be close together as the end is coming?" He was discharged, and I never found out what they did.

Welcome to the world of being a doctor. Alida wants you to listen carefully to the messages behind the information, like a family doctor would listen.

Here's some more advice about relating to patients. The patient can always imagine the situation to be worse than it is. You may think that nothing could be worse than telling someone that they have a cancer which is difficult to treat and they are likely to die from that cancer. But the patient thinks, "I'm going to die from this cancer and I'm going to be in agony from pain at the end." So, you need to anticipate what could be worse than what you are about to tell them and make sure you let them know that you can handle their worst case scenario. "I don't really expect this cancer to be producing much pain, but if it does, we have plenty of options to treat it. I've never had a patient who 'suffered' at the end. It has always been possible to find a way to avoid that." And that has always been true, so I'm comfortable with that statement. And ask them what their concerns are after you are done. We will talk more later about delivering bad news. One thing you need to do is avoid leaving the impression that you are anxious to leave. With your composed posture, let them know that you are available, right now or in the future, to answer any concerns that they may have. I usually end with something like, "Let's finish the tests, get our consultants in here and find out what the treatment options are. Then you and I will talk (or 'we'll all talk' if family is present) and decide the best way to approach this."

Speaking of pain, I have had the good fortune to know and observe several excellent pain specialists. All of them share one important feature. They do not become involved in the anxiety of their patient. I have learned from these devoted specialists that anxiety over the inability to control pain is a major factor in the patient's experience. All of these specialists show great empathy for their patients' pains and all of them maintained a studied, calm demeanor while letting their patient know that they will certainly be able to help with the pain and keep it under control. They show no hint of anxiety.

Must we, as doctors, always tell the truth? Let's start with an easy answer. It is never OK to lie. Never. Now, I personally think that it is perfectly fine to avoid the truth if the patient doesn't want to hear it. They'll usually let you know what they want to hear if you are sensitive to it.

Often, the initial encounter raises concern of a bad diagnosis, or even a high probability of a bad diagnosis, but almost never provides you with certainty of a bad diagnosis. You must learn to use that uncertainty to your patient's advantage. Provide information without your differential diagnosis at first. Just outline the facts. Ask them if they understand. Ask them if they have any questions. If they give you a short no, then they aren't ready to hear what they expect you to say. However, if there are going to be tests, or consultants, who diagnose and treat that bad diagnosis that you are considering, then it is usually better to introduce the concerning diagnosis whether they want to hear it or not because the consultants will (How can they avoid it?) and it may not be in the manner that you, as their current treating physician, would want.

So, similar to what we discussed above, I might say something like, "We can see why your leg is becoming weak. The CT scan shows that there is something on the right side of your brain, gently touching the region on their head. We can't tell exactly what it is right now, we're going to need more tests. Even though I'm not sure what this is, I am concerned that it is something growing that looks like a tumor. It could be an infection but it is possible that it is a cancer, either starting in your brain or coming from some other part of your body. We really won't know until all of the tests are completed. There are a lot of possibilities"

The way I think of this is that, first of all, I really don't know. There were two cases at Einstein in the last couple of years that everyone thought was a glioblastoma multiforme but the neurosurgeon and I were uncertain and kept telling the patient so. These two turned out to be Listeria infections. The truth is that you cannot establish a certain diagnosis from imaging. By including infection, "or other treatable conditions such as inflammation." in my differential for the patient, they gain some time to explore their future. They hear the word cancer, they know what that means. In my imagination, as they try to fall asleep that night, they are considering the prospect of having cancer but can take refuge in the idea "but he said it might be a treatable infection." I think of it as a safe house, for now, to help them avoid panic. Then, as additional test results come in, you can share them, along with a sense of the probability (but not yet certainty), that this might be cancer. But they can still hope. If the final biopsy result does in fact reveal cancer, a week later, at least they have had the opportunity to acclimate to that notion. And maybe it will be Listeria or sarcoid.

One more last topic. I believe that it is important to have an explicit purpose in your mind as you enter the patient's room. What is the purpose of this visit? What do you need to accomplish? That may sound strange to you but there are many purposes to a visit. Diagnosis, treatment options, response to treatment, side effects, new symptoms, sharing second opinions, feedback on lab work, electrophysiology or imaging, helping the caregiver cope, dealing with secondary depression, placement in long term care, on and on.

Sometimes, on the ward, the students and residents have already done a great job of diagnosis and selecting an effective treatment strategy. I might play a more specific role of motivating the patient to comply with these recommendations or to modify an unhealthy lifestyle or just to provide emotional support. Throughout my visit I am aware of that purpose and am setting up and looking for the right opportunity to make my point, to play my role in our team's effort, if you will.

An implicit goal of every visit, however, is that I want my patient to feel good about the visit when we are parting. I want them to know they were heard, to have confidence in me as a physician, to know that I care about them personally and to know that I will help monitor their progress and to help with new conditions that may arise. Except under very rare circumstances, I try to end with a touch of humor, usually based on something that happened during the visit that is ending. Base it on some event, some silly statement, some *faux pas* on my part or their part or by a family member or the resident who is with me. It's my attempt at providing a human touch, putting a cap on the business that was addressed, and leaving off with a light mood so they will look forward to the next visit. Anyway, that's my goal and that's how I remember Dr. Bradley ending his visits as he escorted the patient back to the waiting room for their checkout, gently smiling and sharing some pleasantry.

Chapter 9. Prognosis (Predicting Outcome)

In this chapter we will discuss several topics related to prognosis or, more correctly, predicting outcome for patients, including the use of the Rankin Score to communicate the predicted outcome after cardiac arrest. Prognosis is usually discussed after a major medical event, such as severe trauma, life-threatening infection, the diagnosis of cancer or systemic autoimmune disease, attempted suicide or a major vascular event such as a cardiac arrest. Prognosis is rarely considered for a cold or chronic medical conditions such as hypertension or osteoarthritis even though it is logically possible to do so.

What is prognosis? Prognosis is, strictly speaking, the natural history of the disease. This was a prized art of physicians a long time ago but fell into disfavor when antibiotics and other successful treatments were discovered. What we usually mean when we discuss prognosis is the predicted outcome, including treatment.

Strictly speaking, the prognosis for herpes simplex virus encephalitis has not changed in the last 50 years, it is still likely that the patient will die of the disease if untreated. So, whether you treat the patient or not, the natural history is that the patient will die. But there have been dramatic advances in treatment and the predicted outcome of HSVE over the years. It is literally the difference between life and death whether you do or don't treat the patient. But the natural history, strictly speaking, has not changed.

Of course, now a days, if someone asks your opinion about the prognosis, they actually are asking you to predict the patient's outcome, taking into account treatment options.

Sometimes, however, the question of prognosis as natural history is actually relevant. Consider, for example, a patient with metastatic brain mets. The question of how aggressive to be diagnosing and treating the mets hinges upon the expected survival of the patient. In the absence of good systemic treatment options, which is, thankfully, becoming less common, the prognosis for survival with that cancer is a key question that guides our approach to the apparent brain mets.

A similar situation may arise in other conditions. For example, a carotid endarterectomy or stent for carotid stenosis should only be considered if the patient has a life expectancy of at least 2.5 years because complications associated with the procedures actually favor conservative treatment if the patient doesn't survive at least that long. After 2.5 years, however, the reduced rate of stroke recurrence due to the procedure makes the early risk worth it in the long run. For a patient with severe heart disease in whom all useful therapies have been exhausted, given the risk of the procedure, it may make sense to opt for conservative medical management.

There is no such thing as a procedure without complications. While "a chance to cut is a chance to cure" is often true, every procedure has a measurable complication rate. Therefore, when compared to conservative medical management, on average, it is usually the case that the surgically treated patients will do less well immediately after the procedure. However, assuming the procedure confers a long-term benefit over medical management, eventually, at some point, the surgically treated patients will be better off.

It is important to become familiar with this general concept and how to explain it to your patients. Basically, in principle, the patient would be accepting a higher early risk in exchange for long-term benefit if they select the procedure. The concepts apply not only to surgical or interventional procedures but also to very complex modern medical regimens such as bone marrow replacement, gene therapy and CAR-T cell therapies. Patients need to learn about both the qualitative and quantitative aspects of the proposed procedure and the conservative management. We discussed these matters related to decision making. How severe are the disease consequences? How great is the benefit in the long run for treating the disease? How high is the risk of a complication? How severe are the procedural complications? Sometimes, you will know the answers to these questions. However, in our increasingly complex and rapidly changing medical environment, it often requires the involvement of one or more consultants to get these answers accurately. When this is the case, I promise the patient that I will function as their primary care doctor through the decision making process. I will listen to the consultants with them, help them to ask the right questions, and then sit with them and their family to help them decide on the course of action that is best for them. Note that this process helps me learn as well.

A Uniquely Modern Dilemma

Recent developments that permit increasingly accurate prognosis and increased specificity for patient management have created a unique dilemma.

It is often the case that the consultants will need more information to answer the above questions. More tests may be wanted to understand the prognosis of the patient before deciding on a procedure or complex medical regimen. This was originally referred to as "personalized medicine" but it is now simply accepted that the genetics of a cancer or a host of other factors may modify the recommendations of sub-specialists. Over time I have noticed an unintended down side to this approach. Obtaining the information necessary to optimize the treatment recommendations can take so long that the patient progresses to a worse functional status during the workup. I have seen patients with complex conditions progress to the point that their quality of life becomes unacceptable to them while awaiting treatment recommendations. No doubt, our workups will improve with time so that even complex conditions will be evaluated expeditiously. Until then, however, this is a factor which you must navigate with your consultants and patients.

Do Not Lose Sight of the Forest

There are times when a consultant may be asked for a prognosis (prediction of outcome) regarding a specific issue and they fail to look at the patient as a whole. The consultant feels that the specific condition is manageable but fails to take into account the fact that the patient′s underlying medical conditions makes the management of the specific condition much more complicated and less effective, as well as result in a markedly shortened life expectancy and impaired functional status.

If that is true, then why was the consultant brought in to begin with? Sometimes there is no good answer, it should not have happened. Sometimes, the referring team wants some conservative recommendations that can be accomplished within the limitations of the patient's overall condition. Of course, without a prior conversation between the referrer and consultant, it is unlikely that the nuances of the consult request will be addressed optimally.

If the consultant misses the big picture but is smart enough to speak with the referring team before sharing too much information with the patient and family, then little harm is done in missing the big picture.

The real problem arises if the consultant speaks to the patient and family before becoming aware of the big picture. In that case, they may pass along a prognosis that is unrealistic and overly optimistic. The referring team, or the consultant, then has to modify the prior comments and re-educate the family about the bigger picture, etc. Not good. The family hears conflicting messages and, not surprisingly, loses confidence in the entire treating team.

This scenario reinforces the idea that it is best for consultants to work closely with the referring team and to avoid excessive discussion with the patient and family until their opinions have been integrated into the big picture through discussion.

Using the Rankin Scale to Convey Prognosis

I love the Rankin Scale. It has been the outcome metric of most stroke research since 1995 but it also can be extraordinarily useful in organizing your thinking about prognosis. While I use the Rankin

Scale, there are many other useful ordinal functional outcome scales that can be applied in the same manner. Let's proceed using the Rankin Scale for now though.

First of all, here is my simple version of the scale that should be easy to remember:

Rankin 0 - Normal, no deficits

Rankin 1 - There is a deficit but no disability (Think mild facial palsy)

Rankin 2 - There is a disability but the patient is able to carry on a normal lifestyle (Think about someone using a cane but continuing to work, care for themself, have a happy home life)

Rankin 3 - There is a disability, the patient requires assistance with some activities of daily living (ADL's) (Think about not being able to button your shirt or put on your shoes, or requiring help to get in and out of the shower or a car)

Rankin 4 - Major disability, all or nearly all ADL's require assistance, ambulation is difficult or lost

Rankin 5 - The patient requires 24/7 nursing care, they may be conscious or not

Rankin 6 - Dead

Notice that the Rankin scores define three groups. Patients who are Rankin 0-2 are all independent. After a major event such as stroke, head trauma or cardiac arrest, all of these can be considered "Good Outcomes."

Conversely, Rankin 5 and 6, are "Bad Outcomes." In an old study, 73% of Americans would rather be dead than Rankin 5. That is why those two scores are often combined prior to statistical analysis since ordinal scales must be monotonic for valid analysis and that assumption would be violated if 5 is worse than 6. At any rate, you get it, Rankin 5 and 6 are bad.

Rankin 3 and 4 are "in between." They're not "Bad", but they're not "Good." This group requires a bit more explanation. First of all, there is a big difference between 3 and 4. Secondly, there are good 3's and bad 3's, good 4's and bad 4's. The functional categories are very wide. Thirdly, most families can see the motor deficits of 3's and 4's but fail to appreciate that there are usually cognitive deficits and personality changes that are associated with these states, especially with Rankin 4. So the family sees only the need to help their loved one overcome the motor deficits and they are eager to do that. But they fail to appreciate that their loved one may be a very, very different person than before the event, possibly minimally interactive. It is, therefore, important that anticipated cognitive and personality deficits become an explicit part of the prognosis.

Communicating Predicted Outcome After Cardiac Arrest Using the Rankin Scale

The Rankin Score is particularly useful for communicating the predicted outcome of a cardiac arrest patient to the family and to the referring team. The question is, how do you summarize your prognosis after accounting for all of the available data? Let's put our knowledge and experience of Bayesian reasoning to work. Do you think you could summarize a patient's prognosis with a single percentage point estimate? Obviously not. You would attempt to describe the most probable outcome but include possible less likely outcomes, with some indication of the likelihood for each. In other words, you would develop a distribution of probable outcomes.

This is where the Rankin Scale becomes helpful. The best way I know to illustrate the prognosis after cardiac arrest, or other severe event that landed the patient in the ICU, is to create a histogram with 7 categories, from Rankin 0 to 6 on the horizontal axis and your estimate of the probability that the patient will achieve each of the possible scores within the next 3 months on the vertical scale. As always, the sum of all categories must equal 100%.

Let's take a common example and create our estimate.

The patient is a 78 year old white male with long-standing CHF. He has been hospitalized twice in the last year and requires home O_2. He complained to his family of severe shortness of breath for a couple of hours and then became abruptly unresponsive and slumped in his chair. Family began CPR, EMS arrived in 7 minutes, ROSC was achieved in the ED with a total time to ROSC of 32 minutes. He had brief myoclonic seizures controlled when propofol was started for sedation after intubation. His initial CT scan was probably unremarkable although the gray-white differentiation was questionably blurred, EEG was not yet available, his creatinine had risen to 2.3 within 12 hours and his hepatic transaminases are slightly elevated. His ejection fraction on bedside ECHO is 20%. He is now off sedation but not arousing.

Now, it is likely that you have never done this type of exercise before but watch how intuitive it is. If I ask you, what is the probability that this patient will achieve a Rankin 0 within the next 3 months, that is completely back to normal. What will you say? You will look at me skeptically and say "0." And you would be right. What about Rankin 1? "0." Rankin 2? "Sorry, it's still 0."

Let's take a step back and look at the big picture before going further. What just happened? You have just excluded the possibility that this patient will achieve independence at 3 months. Justifiably! In the next chapter on difficult discussions, we will return to this example. For now, I just want to point out that you are already well on your way to being able to estimate prognosis in a manner that is useful for the family. Taking future independence off the table with near certainty is a big deal!

Let's continue and move to the other extreme. Rankin 6? Well, do you believe that this patient is certain to survive this hospitalization? Obviously not. He has a significant risk of dying no matter what treatment is given. Pick a number 0 to 100%. How about 40%? Could be higher, right? What about Rankin 5. Honestly, if he doesn't die, he is extremely likely to end up 24/7 nursing care at 3 months. You know this intuitively. So then, the overwhelming probability is that he is going to have a "bad outcome." This is not what anyone wants to hear but is extremely useful information for the family and referring team.

What about in between with Rankin 3 or 4? It is usually not possible to exclude a Rankin 4 outcome but the probability for this patient would be remote. I would usually estimate 3% for a patient such as this although studies suggest that the result should really be explained as 0% but with confidence limits of 0 to 3%. The actual number doesn't matter, it's small but non-zero. Rankin 3 is probably unrealistic for this patient.

And don't lose sight of the fact that he has severe CHF at baseline that will have a major impact on his outcome and ability to tolerate rehab. Clearly it is worth engaging the family in a discussion of his prior quality of life.

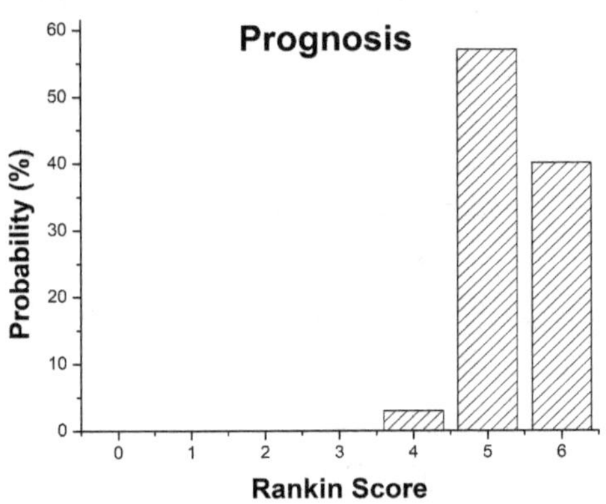

This discussion is usefully summarized by the histogram above. The distribution of outcomes that we estimate is visually obvious and provides the referring doctors with a strong intuitive sense of the prognosis. I frequently drew the histogram in the chart when notes were hand-written. Now its textual and the immediacy and overall distribution is less obvious. So I frequently grab a piece of paper and draw the histogram for the residents on the primary team. The paper gets thrown away but the visual image persists in their minds.

We have considered prognosis after cardiac arrest in some detail and seen how we can summarize the prognosis in a useful manner using a probability histogram of the Rankin Scale. The same techniques can be applied in a wide variety of conditions by changing the outcome scale to suit your specific patient.

Chapter 10. Goals of Care Discussions

This chapter will deal with an important topic that can be a source of considerable stress to doctors at every stage of their career. Not surprisingly, there are a lot of individual skills to learn. It is my goal that, by the end of the chapter, that you will be comfortable helping families deal with the difficult situations associated with life-threatening illnesses in their loved ones.

General Considerations

First, you need to overcome the misconception that this is, somehow, different than everything else that you learn in medicine. It isn't different, it is the same. To emphasize the point, I often say that you should approach this the same way you would learn to start an IV. Running a Goals of Care (GoC) discussion involves a series of technical skill that you learn! Yes, it is complicated, and requires compassion and empathy, but so does nearly everything else that you do as a doctor. You will be much more effective if you approach GoC meetings as a technical skill in the same sense as everything else.

It goes without saying that every GoC situation is different. The disease, the patient, the family and the point in the hospitalization are all important factors in determining how to proceed. Of course, this has been true for every page of this book. While everything in this chapter pertains to a critically ill patient, some aspects may not apply to your particular patient and so every recommendation that follows is implicitly followed by the phrase "if appropriate."

Most GoC meetings have 6 discrete sections:

- Preparation
- Opening
- Review of patient status and related questions
- Prognosis and related questions
- Discussion, including future management
- Closing

Preparation for the Meeting

Some of the most important practices related to GoC meetings occur prior to the actual meeting. This cannot be overstated and will be addressed in more detail below. In the broadest sense, the meeting begins with the determination by the treating team that a meeting is needed. There may or may not have been a sentinal event that requires a face to face meeting. It may simply "be time" to bring the family up to date. Occasionally, the family requests a meeting. Usually the meeting is initiated by the primary team but it could be suggested by a consultant or the ICU nurse. At that point, the key members who should be present need to be contacted to determine their availability and then the family is contacted to select from the available date/time options. It is usually the ICU nurse or a junior resident who contacts the family but this may vary among medical centers and individuals. In many centers, that liaison role is addressed by a social worker. Occasionally it may be a member of the hospital chaplaincy. There is often a friendly "negotiation" among all involved staff, headed by the nurse, social worker or other coordinator, to identify the optimal time for staff and family.

Finally, a meeting time and place are made known to all participants. The "where" is usually in an ICU family conference room or other nearby meeting room. Depending on the number of family/friends who want to attend, larger spaces may be needed. On rare occasions, meetings may be held out of doors to handle an unusually large group. In the current era, it is not unusual for some people to attend remotely by computer. When a computer is going to be used, a staff member needs to be responsible to send the invitation to one family member who then shares it with those who will attend remotely. A staff member familiar with the computer and meeting software should ensure that everything is running properly prior to the start of the meeting. However, I am NOT a fan of remote attendance and I am not shy about sharing that with family members. There are times when long distances make it necessary however.

In addition, arrangements must be made to account for a larger number of family members than is permitted by hospital policy during standard visiting hours. Also, it needs to be established who will guide the family members to the conference room if it is in the ICU or in a difficult to find location. It's not a bad idea to check out the conference room right before bringing in the first visitors to clean up food and other items as well as to set up the remote video streaming service.

All staff members who will participate in the meeting should meet beforehand, as a group if possible. At that brief meeting, usually conducted informally outside the patient's room or the nursing station, everyone should agree on the specific purpose(s) and goal(s) of the meeting, the key messages that are to be conveyed to the family and how this will be coordinated. If any procedures or other treatment are almost certain to be needed for patient management, then all team members should be made aware of that fact.

Several operational issues should be addressed prior to joining the meeting. Who is responsible for leading the meeting? Who will present each major piece of information? Who will respond to the family's questions about the major concerns? Usually it is clear from each team member's specialty but there are often unique features that may modify that guideline. Also, it is not uncommon for one team member to lead the early phase of the meeting but plan to transfer facilitation of the discussion to a second team member at some agreed upon transition point.

<u>Immediately</u> before the meeting, at least one team member should re-examine the patient and speak with the treating nurse to establish that there have been no sudden or unexpected changes in the patient's status. If there has been a change, all team members should be notified of the changes before joining the meeting. I don't need to tell you how embarrassing it is if a team member provides information or recommendations that are no longer accurate or appropriate, and how severely that damages the family's confidence in the entire team.

It is important to know in advance who has the patient's health care power of authority (POA) since they will play a unique role in current and future discussions. You will find that the POA is not always the person making decisions for the patient. The POA may acknowledge this openly or it may simply be *de facto*. If the patient has not declared a POA in a will or other signed, notarized legal document, then there are state laws that determine who fulfills the role of POA. In Pennsylvania, the spouse is given priority if no one has been named in advance, followed by adult children, parents and adult siblings. It is a good idea to obtain the help of the hospital legal department to establish POA status when it is not completely clear due to prior marriages, common law marriages or other complicating circumstances.

And make sure that all team members know each other's names before the meeting. A member may be distracted or not present during the introductions. You will be referring to each other for additional input during the meeting or to reiterate each other's roles. The family wants to know that you are a single, organized team!

What is the Purpose of the Meeting?

The importance of establishing the purposes and goals of the meeting before the meeting starts has already been emphasized. Clearly, the purposes and goals of each meeting will vary with the specific circumstances. The following discussion relates to a specific relatively common situation. It is assumed for the rest of this discussion that this is the first formal meeting with the extended family for an older patient who is critically ill, typically 24-48 hours after admission to ICU. It is likely that earlier small and informal meetings with key family members have already taken place with the first encounter occurring on admission to obtain history and address emergency issues. It is likely that there already have been bedside updates for key family members as well. These early meetings are characterized by uncertainty, emergent actions related to stabilizing the patient, as well as orienting the family and establishing early relationships.

Understand that the purpose and specifics of the meeting could be very different depending on the patient and the disease involved. The patient may be much younger, the mother of a newborn, the family bread winner or might even be a child. Younger patients have a much greater ability to recover from catastrophic injuries than older patients so that prognosis has to be much more conservative. Also, the patient may have been relatively healthy immediately prior to an unexpected presenting event or this event may have been anticipated for some time. Family dynamics may differ dramatically, possibly involving adolescent children or siblings, or the parents of the patient. All of these factors and many others besides have important impact on the specifics of the meeting.

Starting the Meeting

GoC meetings may trickle to a start or begin all at once. Sometimes doctors, nurses, staff and family are all at the bedside and you all walk together to the conference room. Sometimes, family members arrive and are seated and staff arrive over a few minutes. Sometimes you wait awhile for the last family member to arrive.

Where should you sit? I like to sit away from the door, in a spot where I cannot get out until the family opens a path. That may sound a bit dangerous but it has never led to any problem. Instead, I believe that it sends an important non-verbal message that says to the family that I am not anxious or afraid of them but rather that we are all together in this. Furthermore, it establishes that I am going to stay with them until they are satisfied that all of their needs have been met. I cannot suddenly get up and walk out.

The meeting begins formally when the staff leader introduces themself and suggests that we go around the table giving our names and relationship to the patient. Around the table we go, usually clockwise and including any second row or standing room people, without regard to relationship as family or staff. "My name is Sarah and I am his mother". My name is Dr. Jones and I am the first year resident on his primary team."

Occasionally, the ICU attending, who is the Attending of record, may be occupied by emergencies and cannot participate in the meeting. When that is true, it is appropriate for the team's most senior resident or fellow to apologize to the family on behalf of the Attending with appropriate explanation. This should then be followed by "Of course we will make Dr. Jones aware of everything that goes on at this meeting. That's important because Dr. Jones is the doctor who is actually responsible for Mr. Harris." Consultants who are participating in the meeting will usually reiterate that point when they speak, "after discussion with Dr. Jones." The family needs to know that we are a team with clear chain of command.

Usually, the next step is for the agreed upon staff leader to provide a brief description of the purpose of the meeting and a brief outline of the meeting to come as already discussed during preparation. This usually includes an indication of which other staff members are going to present information and what information they will present.

Finally, in my opinion, for this first meeting, if at all possible, the leader should indicate that we will <u>not</u> be requiring any decisions of the family today, that the purpose of this meeting is for us to present information and for them to ask questions. There are many reasons that I recommend this. After all, we are assuming that this is a first meeting. Unless there is urgent need for some management decisions, which is uncommon, it is better to begin in this manner. Why is it better?

Most importantly, if the family is expecting a negative recommendation or demand for "decision", they will be continuously arguing in their mind against everything we say during the conference, focusing on the exceptions instead of the rules and "defending" their loved one against our expected hasty judgements. We don't want that. On the other hand, if you take early decision-making off the table at the beginning of the meeting, then they will immediately relax and listen intently to what you have to say. They can comfortably explore the meaning of our information regarding their loved one. That is exactly what we want.

Secondly, there simply may not be enough information available for recommendations or judgements on our part or theirs. You know this at the start but they don′t. This is just a first meeting. The idea is to build a foundation of shared information and relationships for the future. During this meeting you will be able to indicate the information that will be used for further diagnosis and monitoring of the patient so that future family updates have meaning within the context created during this first meeting.

Third, later in the meeting we are going to counsel the family not to make any "decisions" for the patient. What? Yes, that is my primary goal in this type of meeting. That will make more sense later in this chapter when we get there.

Sharing Information

One important aspect of nearly every GoC meeting is the sharing of information. This is a two way street!

The medical team needs to provide the information that the family needs in order to understand the current situation. That involves a review of the major events that lead up to the current situation. It will help the family to be able to trace a story beginning with the patient's past medical history, onset of acute illness prior to calling EMS, during transport, upon arrival in the ED and since admission, based on our current information. If the patient had presented with trauma, then the PMH may have less importance and our understanding of the trauma and related injuries much more emphasis but the process is similar. The information should be presented in a straightforward manner. Avoid, for the moment, distracting discussion of issues that the family is likely to raise. These are typically of a "what if" nature and "why didn't" scenarios. Simply say that these are important questions and that there will be time to address those issues later "if you like" but "for now it's important that we all have a clear picture of what has happened."

Stick to the facts at this stage. After the information has been presented, the discussion leader should pause the meeting and ask if there are any questions "about what has been said so far." There will often be questions from the family about issues not yet discussed such as next steps and prognosis. Again, the response to those should be, "That is a really important question, but let's hold that for now. I just want to be sure right now that we have been clear in presenting the information to this point so that we are all on the same page." Note that we don't ask if they understand but rather if we have been clear. It is our responsibility to be sure that our presentation has been intelligible for everyone. We are not testing their learning skills.

It is appropriate and easy to include the patient's earlier and current treatments during this phase of information sharing, along with a sense of how the patient has responded to the treatments. In addition, any immediately imminent medical management or minor procedures such as arterial lines, etc., can also be presented in this phase. Rather than getting into potential procedural complications at this point, however, I would just tell them, if they ask, that we will be obtaining informed consent and that will include "all of the details involved, including why we are recommending it and the risk of complications." Unless it is nearly certain that some major procedure will be needed, such as neurosurgery, abdominal organ repairs or cardiac procedures, those major procedures can be left for later in the meeting or another meeting altogether. Similarly, unless dialysis or other restorative procedures are nearly certain, discussion of those also can be avoided or, if very likely, they can be mentioned as possible treatments that may be discussed at follow-up meetings, "since we are not sure if they will be needed."

This is a good opportunity for another pause. Before asking family if there are more questions, I like to obtain additional input from other staff members regarding the information that already has been presented or that is closely related. I usually just turn to the other members and ask "Have I left anything out? Anything else that you want to add at this point?" Continue to keep the family focused on the medical facts thus far and the near future. You can indicate that "we're going to discuss his prognosis and our recommendations shortly" if that will help. Questions from the family generally about facts and our presentation flow naturally at this point. They are getting a sense of how the meeting operates.

It is now time to get some input from the family. This has two obvious purposes. First, we need information about the patient's past medical history and how their disease has affected their pre-morbid (ie - prior to the admitting event) functional status and quality of life. For example, it is not at all clear from the fact that "Dementia" is listed in a patient's medical record what that means for the patient or family. It might mean he forgets names at times or it might mean that he wanders around the house at night keeping everyone awake, elopes on occasion and had set the kitchen on fire a couple of months ago. Or anything in between. The same is true of "CHF", "COPD", "arthritis" and any other symptom complex.

It is usually best to begin with an open ended set of questions. "You know your father much better than we do. It would be really helpful if you could give us a sense of what he was like. How did he spend his days? What did he like to do? Were any of his medical problems limiting his activities?" From there on, just engage the family in a discussion that allows them to create a picture of your patient. They may make you aware of things that you later share with other staff members to help them see this patient as a person in their pre-morbid state. It's hard to tell a "saint" from a "sinner" with a critically ill patient in the ICU. It helps to know who you are caring for. The family's information may also have major impact on prognosis or on the eventual management judgements that are intrinsic to GoC discussions for critically ill patients, including how the pre-morbid functional status may limit treatment options.

The patient's personality is a major part of this sharing from the family. Was the patient "a fighter," or chronically depressed, or "couldn't stand doctors." Reflect on this latter statement, which is not uncommon. Should a patient who avoided doctors their whole life be forced to endure months or years of medical care now that they are incapacitated and can't speak for themselves? That is clearly relevant information for later GoC discussions.

You will also learn a great deal about family relationships while the family is speaking about the patient. Who are the key players? What is the structure of the family? Who is an ally in keeping the GoC discussion on task and who will be disruptive?

You also need to learn how the patient feels about intensive care and surviving with potentially severe disabilities in case things develop in that direction. So, if the family doesn't present that information on their own, you need to ask if the patient had previously expressed how he would feel about being this sick. "Has he ever spoken about how he felt watching other friends or family members who were in a similar situation?" The Palliative Care team or a social worker will always ensure this is addressed.

Prognosis

The technical aspects of estimating prognosis were addressed in the last chapter. Here we discuss the role of predicting outcome within the GoC discussion as well as reiterate a few key aspects of prognosis. We are still discussing the first family meeting of a critically ill patient in the ICU.

If it hasn't already been stated, I begin prognosis by stating the obvious. "Obviously, he is critically ill or he wouldn't be in the ICU." After a very brief pause, I then add "When I say critically ill, I mean that he is not completely stable. Things seem stable right now, but they can change very quickly. He can get much sicker very quickly if any additional problems develop." I'd avoid the word "complications" since that can carry the connotation of iatrogenic error for some people and that is not what we mean. "Problems" seems better suited.

The point of this last statement is that you need to let them know that the patient's survival is not a certainty. It is always sad when a less experienced, optimistic well-meaning staff member focuses heavily on the best possible path forward and best outcomes in order to encourage the family. It's natural enough, I have done this myself. But the simple truth is that critically ill patients are unstable and things can "turn sour" with little warning. That includes fatal secondary events such as pulmonary emboli or sepsis. When the prior information and prognosis to the family has been consistently optimistic, and there has been no such warning, then the family is seriously disturbed if the worst does occur. "No one told us he was that sick. What happened, what went wrong?" They mean "What did you do wrong?" So, you must let them know that this is a possibility. I usually say something like "You need to know that even though he is stable right now, things can change quickly when a patient is as sick as he is. It is not even certain that he is going to survive." You will feel and see the shockwave travel through the family when you say this. So I immediately use my hands to create the modified stop sign as discussed in earlier chapters, and quickly add, "We don't expect this, but you need to know that it is a possibility." As you can imagine, you now have their close attention for the rest of the discussion of prognosis.

The next step is to address his expected functional status using the Rankin scale related techniques discussed in the previous chapter. It may be premature to actually offer even an estimate of the prognosis at this point, however. That's ok, almost better for the family. Instead, in that case, we simply tell them it is too early and lay out the foundation of predicting functional outcomes, Good, Bad and In-between, as discussed in detail in the last chapter. I also review the information that we will be using to provide them with an estimate. I let them know that we never have certainty, especially since we don't yet know "the full extent of what injury to his brain and other organs has already occurred." I go on to say "There is no crystal ball. But I want you to understand the kind of information that we use to try to predict his outcome." I then review the key points, of the type we have already discussed, organized around the relevant clinical, lab, electrophysiology and imaging data categories and let them know which information we are already following or will be following. I also tell them that we will share all of that information, "good or bad", as it becomes available. Then I review the information that we already have and let them know what is good and what is not good. For example, "The average cardiac arrest patient at Einstein regains their own heart beat after 22 minutes. Your father didn't regain his until 30 minutes." I don't even draw a conclusion from that, it's obvious. "But, his first head CT in the ED didn't show any evidence of injury, so that's good. It's just too early to tell how he's going to do yet." The family is usually almost relieved to hear that.

I sometimes pause at this point and make the relationship between staff and family a bit more transparent. "We feel that we don't have the right to withhold information from you. So, whether its good news or bad news, we are going to share new information with you as it becomes available. We'll also give you a sense of what it means to us and how it might push our management recommendations one way or another." Families are nearly always comfortable with this type of relationship. They want good news of course but they know that they need to deal with bad news if that's the reality. We have already given them a sense that some things may be out of our control and that injury may already have occurred prior to the beginning of our management. It is important that they understand this before any formal prognosis is offered.

Next is to clarify or re-state the future crucial breakpoints in the patient's status that would alter the prognosis. "We need to keep his seizures under control. If we take away the anesthetics that he is on and he starts seizing again even though he is on three seizure medicines, that would be very concerning. We're all watching him and we will keep the EEG running to monitor him. But that would be very serious as I don't know what else we could do for him." The same kind of information is presented for each organ. He needs to come off the four pressors he is on, we might need to recommend dialysis, he may need additional abdominal surgeries, his foot may need to be amputated. We also have to help them begin to deal with uncertainty like we do by giving them a sense of what "is probably going to happen" or "might happen" or "isn't likely to happen but we're still not sure." Medicine is the art of probability.

It might be appropriate to indicate potential complications that are common as a result of our current or anticipated management. (For this purpose, "complication" is appropriate.) Again, let them know how we are monitoring the patient and what that would mean if the complication does arise. "We'll keep giving you regular updates on his progress."

We also need to give them a sense of how the passage of time affects prognosis. "The most important thing is for him to wake up. As we've discussed, he is in a coma right now. While there is no hard cutoff, it's obvious that the longer he stays in a coma the less likely he is to wake up or return to his former self. Each day is important. We'll let you know if we are seeing signs that he is arousing. It also would be helpful for us if you could tell us if you see any signs that he is waking up. You know him better than we do." You might add, if appropriate to his injury, "I'd feel a lot better if he wakes up in the next couple of days." That would be appropriate after cardiac arrest or metabolic coma but might not be after head injury or if the patient is expected to remain on anesthetic agents as part of his pulmonary management. I usually also add, "You know, not just that. You are part of the team keeping an eye on him, so if you notice anything that doesn't seem right or that you don't understand, then you should say something or ask. Your input is welcome and we like questions. You can just mention it to his nurse (pointing to him/her)."

I'm not eager to introduce any time constraints at our first meeting, those are best left for later meetings but sometimes the family asks about how long we think we should "watch" the patient. Most of the time, the initial family response is going to be conservative, they want as much time as possible. However, in some cases, they are aware that the patient had been suffering and had anticipated this event, even was eager for it. The family already has a sense of the devastating nature of the injury and they know that his medical condition is only going to get worse. In that case, the family may really be asking "How long do we have to wait to be respectful, or "legal," before we can end his misery.

Which is why information sharing is a two way street.

Goals of Care

The term "Goals of Care" basically signifies a series of judgements about the long term care of an individual who has experienced a disease or suffered an injury severe enough to require admission to the ICU and in whom the prognosis includes a relatively high probability of death or permanent loss of independence. How high? High enough that his patient care team believes that there is need to discuss this with the family to determine if the patient would want to survive with this level of disability.

Note that, right from the very definition, this is about what the patient would want. This is critical to the process!

Even my first experiences with GoC made it obvious that there is a major problem having the family make a decision for the patient because it is almost inevitable that, sooner or later, some or all of the family members will experience a sense of guilt. If life support measures are withheld, then the family feels guilty because they "gave up too soon." If life support measures are continued and the patient survives but is still in a nursing home 3 months later, unable to care for themself, having to be cleaned by nurses from urine and feces throughout the day, requiring intermittent procedures for trach, PEG or urinary retention, or frequent hospitalizations for UTI's or pneumonias, then they inevitably ask themselves "What did we do? Why did we put him through this?"

This struck me as a cruel insult to add to the wound of losing their loved one. So, literally from my first encounters as a resident onward, the elimination of guilt among family members has been among my top priorities in these discussions. Over the years, I have come to believe that it is actually impossible for one person to make a decision for another person. That should not be the family's role, we should not ask that of them. But when I tell them that, they immediately respond, "Well, obviously, he can't answer so what are you saying?" What I am saying, to you the reader, is that we act most ethically when we do what the patient would want us to do given the current information. That's the only answer I know. So I tell the family, "If we do this right, it won't be about what you would want for yourself, and certainly not what I would do if it were me. Your role is not to decide for him, but to be his advocate. We need to think about what he would want us to do in this circumstance and then you ask us to do that. You need to be his advocate so that we follow his wishes." These are very powerful words in a GoC discussion. The discussion is now re-focused in an entirely new direction.

I introduce this concept in the very first GoC discussion. Now you can see the value of telling them that we are not going to make a decision today. In fact, we are never going to make a decision. We are all going to try to figure out what the patient would want. You can also see the value of getting to know the patient's personality, his attitude to doctors and his expressed opinions about others in a similar situation. You obtained that information before this topic was introduced so that it is a more "unbiased" evaluation from the family. By the way, when I use the word family, I am implicitly including close friends.

You rarely need to ask any questions to facilitate this discussion, it just bursts forth. One or more family members are usually eager to express their opinion. As you can imagine, there is nearly an infinite number of possible responses by the family as a whole. You already know that, at this meeting, you won't be "making a decision" so the staff members mainly become observers and facilitators of this part of the discussion among family members. Let everyone speak.

Consider asking someone who hasn't yet spoken for their opinion before the discussion ends. Sometimes, you need to "referee" the discussion to make sure that everyone is heard. This is a difficult time for the family because they are likely to express diverse opinions and there can be reactions to those opinions. Old family differences and rivalries can emerge. "You never even came to visit while he was sick. I've been with him all these last months, not you." *Et cetera.* You need to be ready for this and prepared to smooth these rough waters. Often, there is an older family member, typically not immediate parent or offspring, maybe an uncle or even a brother who can play this role for you. If someone rises to the occasion, let them go, you just sit back and watch. They usually carry "wisdom" with them and they know the family a lot better than you do. In any event, do not get drawn into the fray other than to keep things civil. I find the most useful way of cooling a hot situation, if it arises, is to speak up, get everyone's attention, and say something like, "It is almost always the case that there will be differences at stressful times like this. But everyone loves him and wants what is best for him. So we need to listen to each other and hear what everyone has to say. Getting angry with one another is not going to help find what is best for him. That is what we need to focus on." Note that it isn't always a negative to have these family issues and differences of opinion emerge during the GoC meeting. It's probably better for everyone if those emerge in the more formal hospital setting with observers and "referees" present than at home where there are far fewer restraints. You have to learn to tolerate disagreement but prevent it from creating or worsening animosities. Look, no one said this would be easy, certainly not me.

The Closing

When everyone has spoken, and everyone's sentiments are known, you are ready to begin to draw the meeting to its close. Hopefully, by this time, the family has a good sense of you as a doctor and team and trusts your fairness and honesty.

I begin the close by turning to the person with POA and those that you have observed to be their most valued advisors, and say, "I think its time for us to wind down. We don't need to find any answers today, we don't even have enough information yet, it's too early. Anyway, maybe he'll improve and then we can all just celebrate together. What I am asking though, is for you to begin to discuss what he would want in case things don't go the way we want them to. Sit as a family and think about him. Open your hearts to him. Think about everything you know about him and discuss what he would want. Not what you would want or even what you think would be best. Only what he would want. That's the answer you are looking for. And please, as you do this, remember that all of you love him and want what is best for him. So listen to each other and don't become angry with one another. I would feel terrible if I have been the cause for any hard feelings in your family." Note that I have purposely made them responsible for me by my implied guilt if there are new irreconcilable family rifts. Feelings can be raw after a meeting like this and that leaves them open to understanding what I am saying and it confirms for them that I really do care about them as well as the patient.

I would prefer to avoid DNR questions at this first meeting. This is a bit controversial, not all would agree, but we prefaced the meeting by saying we wouldn't be asking them for decisions and that promise has been a prominent part of the meeting. However, even I would agree that if the patient is unstable or in shock, then it has to be done. If a code is imminent, it is better to ask now than at 3AM. In which case it goes something like this. Usually, the resident on the primary team will squirm visually and murmur out loud. That is my opportunity to say, "I'm sorry to bring this up but Dr. Jones is reminding me that your father is really unstable right now and we are concerned that his heart may stop at any time so there is one thing that we really do need to discuss. If his heart were to stop before our next meeting, should we resuscitate him?" It may be appropriate to add, "My concern is that if his heart stops despite everything that we are doing now, then he is telling us that he is not likely to do well going forward. And I don't want him to suffer unnecessarily." I also let them know that nothing else is going to change. "Of course, even if he is DNR, nothing else changes. We would continue everything that we are doing to keep him alive and bring him back. NOTHING else would change." Stop and gauge their reaction. Often they will just agree, sometimes they will say "We're not ready for that." Sometimes they'll ask to be alone for a few minutes and then they'll give you an answer.

I hope you noticed the phrase "unnecessary suffering." We will return to that shortly but first let's bring this meeting to a close.

I like to end by acknowledging how difficult this has been for them. "I know that this has been very hard to hear but I think that it has been worthwhile because now you have a good sense of how to follow what is happening along with us over the next several days. Also, we have given you a huge amount of information and almost certainly you're going to have some questions. 'What did he say about . . . ?'. Everyone does. We're always here, day and night. You can ask any of us any questions that you may have. If we don't know the answer, we'll find someone who does. You can always start with his nurse. His nurse is the person who is most up to date in his care and always knows how to reach us. And remember, if you see a change, let us know." I would re-iterate which team is primary. I conclude with a very brief review of what is to come in the next 24 hours and the key monitors that we are following. Let them know that we will meet again for updates. Ask if there are any last questions that we haven't addressed and call it to a close. Also ask if there are any key family members who would want to be involved but couldn't make this meeting. I take those missing members very seriously and so always offer to review "all of this information" with them, either at the next meeting or when they arrive. The missing people often take control of the discussions at home even though they have little or no knowledge of all that has been discussed.

This meeting almost certainly lasted in the range of an hour. Was it worth it? Yes, a hundred times over. It will save you many, many hours in the future and, more importantly, is necessary to find the best outcome for your patient.

Notice that we have not raised the question of organ donation. First of all it is premature but there are other reasons which we will address as we move onto how to approach subsequent meetings.

Subsequent Meetings

Almost everything that was said for the first meeting applies to subsequent meetings. Preparation including determination of purpose, the sections of the meeting and the techniques discussed during the meeting all are the same. Therefore, the following will address only the unique features of follow-up meetings.

There are additional purposes that may pertain to subsequent meetings. There may be needed to involve additional family members, or additional positive or negative information has become available that clarifies prognosis, or disease progression has raised the need for additional surgical or restorative procedures, or further clarification of underlying diagnoses has introduced indications for complex managements that have not been discussed previously. A common reason for subsequent GoC meetings is that the patient appears headed for long-term disability and the time is approaching for tracheostomy tube insertion, usually along with a feeding tube. This latter issue forces the question of whether the patient would want to be sustained given the current prognosis and medical/surgical needs.

Based on the above, it is important that preparation ensures that the additional family members and staff, including critical consultants, are involved. All family members whose opinions carry weight, as the POA attempts to forge a consensus, should be present, preferably in person and not online.

Also, you need to be aware of any hidden "non-participant." Every once in awhile you will have heard about "a family member in

California" who no one on the staff has met or spoken to, but who "has some serious concerns about what's going on" based on information from a local family member. You must make every effort to have that family member participate in the meeting even though this type of person would prefer to act only in the background. It is not uncommon for a hidden person such as this to play a major role in family dynamics, usually as a strongly negative influence and disrupter of the healthy process. You can directly address that with the family POA or other close family if you believe there is someone. "I understand there's another family member in California who has some serious concerns. If there is anyone who feels that way, please make sure they join our meeting so we can address those concerns. And if I can help you make them feel more comfortable by speaking with them, please let me know. I'd be glad to help." Sometimes the POA or closest family member who was delegated to have the final say needs help, almost protection, from this dissident. You can help "provide cover for them" if that would be useful to them. Usually they decline, but on occasion it is a blessing to them and they welcome it.

The follow-up meeting begins with introductions as before and then with a brief summary of what was said at the first meeting. If new family members are present, I ask them if they have been brought up to date by the family, if they have any questions or if they need to have any of the important points discussed again. Most of the time, they will like to hear a re-cap from the team. That is always fine with me because some repetition helps everyone in the family to confirm that they understand. As always, time is provided for family members to ask questions related to the facts and to make sure that all staff have given the input that they feel is important.

Then the expressed purpose of the follow-up meeting is introduced. Since this will be quite specific case by case, let's continue with our example of the patient after cardiac arrest. Let's also assume that, as predicted by the prolonged "down time," the patient remains comatose on Day 10 since admission. He had myoclonic seizures from Days 3 to 5. Although they have stopped, his continuous EEG shows a burst suppression pattern with very low voltage baseline even after his anti-seizure medicines have been tapered and all anesthetics have been discontinued for several days. He is in renal failure and has started dialysis. His follow-up CT scan demonstrates significant diffuse cerebral edema. Hepatic synthesis has not yet returned to normal. None of this is good. It is at least 97% likely that he will end up Rankin 5 or 6. While the primary ICU team may choose to handle this alone, it would not be uncommon to have neurocritical care and palliative care consultants participate in the meeting. I assume, just for simplicity of writing the following text, that I have been chosen to lead the meeting during our team preparation but anyone might have that role. The following also heavily reflects my own personal style.

"Thank you for meeting again with us. During the last several days we have a lot of new information which has to do with your father's prognosis. We've been discussing this every day with some of you during the last week but it's time for everyone to come together. You should know that I am a very straightforward person. My father raised me that way, I can't help it. You don't have to wonder 'What did he mean by that.' I speak pretty plainly. {Pause} Don't think I don't care. I do. But you have each other for support and what you need from me is honest information."

They have a sense for what's coming. I review the above new clinical information with them, emphasizing that each of these factors has a strong negative influence on his ability to recover from his cardiac arrest. "We've previously discussed Good, Bad and In-between outcomes. I'm sorry to have to tell you that there is virtually <u>no</u> chance whatsoever that he will ever be independent again and even the In-between is a very long shot. It is overwhelmingly likely that either he will die before he leaves the hospital or that he will remain unconscious for as long as we maintain him." Note that I did not say, "As long as he lives." Given the above information, I need to convey to them that any hope for a better outcome is no longer reasonable.

That level of certainty is not uncommon in the ICU and needs to be made known. However, there are also times when we don't have that level of certainty. When that is the case, we need to be very clear that we are not certain and try to give some non-numeric sense of the probability that the patient will arouse or eventually be able to participate in ADL's. Frequently, independence remains unrealistic even though regaining some ADL's is possible, sometimes even independence remains a real possibility and that should be expressed along with cautious optimism and a sense of how likely that is.

Returning to our example patient's situation, I end by saying "I'm sorry. I know how hard that is to hear. I wish we could have done more." I mean it when I say that.

Expect a long silence for people to reflect. Leave the silence as long as they need. There is no rush to end it. You should not say something simply because you are uncomfortable with their silence. Some family members may be quite demonstrative at this point, some may wail and storm out of the room. That's OK. In fact, it is usually the case that a family member will say "That's ok, she'll be all right" and another family member goes out to comfort the member who left. Then there will be specific questions about the information and prognosis. It helps to have another team member take over, typically palliative care, social work or clergy will say something comforting and appropriate.

Once the dust has settled from that, then I continue, "The problem is that we are now on a time clock. The tube in his throat can't stay in for more than about 2 weeks total because the complication rate becomes too high. Also, we need to provide him with more reliable nutrition and medication than he can get from the tube in his nose."

"Now I warned you that I speak very plainly so please don't be offended as we have this discussion. We've previously spoken about whether he would want to survive under these circumstances. This is why we asked you to consider it earlier. I want you to know that not everyone would want to survive this way. Many reasonable people would not be OK with living this way. They would not want to be maintained artificially with all of this artificial hydration and artificial nutrition and all of these machines. And they would not like the idea of being completely taken care of by someone else. There are others, though, who would be OK with all of that. We need to discuss what Mr. Harris would want. Remember, it's not about us, it is about him. We don't need to have an answer today, but we don't really have much time left before we need to perform the surgery on his neck and belly for the breathing and feeding tube if we are going to do that. The main point I want to share with you right now is that it is not necessary for us to cause him to survive with these artificial methods if he wouldn't want us to. It is OK for us to allow him to die if that is what he would prefer (not "want") and spare him any unnecessary suffering. Either way is ethical and can reflect your love. The question is simply what he would want." Note that I used the word surgery here and that I have also purposefully used the word "artificial" several times. We are not talking about "starving" him. Left to his own devices, without our artificial support, he would simply die.

At the end of this chapter, I will share a story about the term "unnecessary suffering."

Notice that I have not put much emphasis on the medical procedures. In fact, I usually tell the family "You don't need to worry much about medical decisions at this point. The medical choices are really fairly easy once we know how the patient would want to be treated in this situation. That's the hard part that we all need to focus on." But there will likely be some family members as well as some staff that would prefer to know a bit about how we would manage the patient either way. That's fine. So we present both directions.

Continuing all life support measures is the simpler of the two to explain. "We would ask the surgeons to see your father and then, assuming the surgeon thinks the risk is not too great, we would schedule the procedures. After the procedure we would wait until we're sure the feeding tube works properly and then bring his tube feeds to full strength over a day or two. The good part of this is that he will be a lot more comfortable when we remove the tubes from his nose and his throat. Also the tubes are more effective for suctioning or for feeding and giving medications. It should be possible to have him ready for placement in his long term care facility within about 4 days altogether. During that time you would start looking at places to decide which you prefer, we would make the application, put in for insurance approval and then he can be transferred. Again, about 4 days altogether." The family is often surprised at how quickly this can occur so if I see that then I may add, "Well, he's pretty stable now and his medical problems are a lot less active than they were before." Depending on many factors, I might add, "At this point he will be committed to long term survival. There are very few nursing homes who would be willing to discontinue feeding and the other treatments that he might need once he is admitted there." Note that the "long term care" may be a long term acute care (LTAC), a skilled nursing facility (SNF), or a nursing home. If the cause of the patient's coma was trauma, he might qualify for traumatic brain injury (TBI) rehabilitation. The actual disposition would affect the above explanation of course.

Explaining the course if the family believes that he would not want to survive is a bit more delicate although not more complicated. "The first thing to realize is that we will have changed our primary goal. In most medical situations, we always assume that survival is our primary goal. There's no need to say so, it's understood. But sometimes survival is no longer our primary goal. Sometimes our primary goal is to allow our patient to die in comfort and with dignity. Allowing his family to be with him in peace at the end is also important. So all of our care becomes directed toward those goals. We are going to follow him closely and make sure that he is always comfortable and does not suffer. We can nearly always guarantee that, because we can use as much narcotics as we need to in order to ensure that he is comfortable. Honestly, that is rarely an issue. We also want to stop doing things that cause discomfort such as blood work and keeping his IV's going. We also want to stop the treatments that are sustaining him so that we do not prolong the period of dying. We will take away any medications that are not needed for his comfort, we will stop his artificial hydration and feedings. Basically, everything we do will be for his comfort. That would include continuing his seizure medicines for instance since he would be uncomfortable if he started to seize again." If the patient is no longer intubated, then all I would add at this point is to give them a sense of how long. "It's very hard to predict how long he will survive this way, everyone is different. For most patients, though, death comes between 3 and 7 days. It can be longer or shorter but that's the usual range. During that time, we want you to be with him. You can touch him, hold his hand, talk to him, I do. Bring in some music that he likes. People can visit with him and take their farewell. My last piece of advice to you is to forget this illness and his time in the hospital. Just remember the good times."

If the patient is still intubated, then there is the issue of "palliative extubation." All of the discussion regarding comfort measures as in the above paragraph still are useful but now we have to address the process of extubation. "Together we will pick a time to remove the breathing tube in his throat. You can let us know when everyone has had an opportunity to say their farewells. When you are ready, we will remove the tube, watching him carefully to make sure that he does not feel any air hunger or other discomfort. Again, the narcotics, especially morphine, are very effective if we need them. Now I have to tell you that many patients do not die immediately after the tube is removed. Some do die within minutes, some take hours but some can survive for days." I might give them a more narrow estimate if there are factors related to hemodynamic status which might suggest sooner or later. "But we will take care of him for as long as it takes and we will make sure he is comfortable at all times. Also, we understand that he is your loved one. So whenever he does stop breathing and die, we are not going to just whisk him away. We'll let you know, if you aren't here, and keep him here so that you can come and say good-bye. I hope you'll understand that can't be longer than several hours though."

Once again, I would ask for input from everyone else on the medical team. I usually ask if I have been "fair" and whether there is anything else that we feel is important for the family to know at this point. After another request for questions from the family, we then conclude the meeting.

Whichever direction the family is leaning or has requested, if DNR has not previously been established then it is appropriate to discuss that before closing the meeting. I would reiterate that we need to understand "what he would want" in the next few days and that we are still here for further discussion. The family may ask for a few more days to think or see how he does. That's fine, don't resist that if they ask.

The meeting ends with eye contact, hand shakes or elbow bumps as you and the family prefer, often with hugs and tears. I have already told you that I hug. You will nearly always hear "Thank you, doctor, for everything you have done." Then you know that the family is at peace and you have done your job well, whatever their final response.

I always bring the medical team together for a "post mortem" after every GoC meeting. I suppose the pun is intended. That might take place in the hallway right outside of the room. It's OK for the family to see the doctors and nurses speaking with one another. There's nothing unusual or wrong about that. I will wave to any family member who sees us. I like to ask how other team members think it went. What went well and what did not? Was there anything unspoken by the family that somone noticed? I do this because, as I said at the beginning of this chapter, the GoC meeting is a technical skill. Like any other technical skill, we need to learn from every experience. We need to share feedback. We need to learn from our experience as a team so that we are more effective the next time. A GoC meeting is no exception.

A Few Specific Issues

Words matter. We NEVER "withdraw care." I recommend to everyone that you eliminate that phrase from your vocabulary and become sensitized to it. We may "withdraw life support measures" but that doesn't mean that we neglect the needs of the patient once that course of action is underway. As noted above, withdrawing life support measures indicates that there has been a shift in our primary goal from survival to comfort. Naturally, we still have to give attention to his comfort. I look in every couple of hours during the day on my comfort care ICU patients to confirm that there are no signs of discomfort. I trust our nurses but there is no reason that I shouldn't provide additional observations. Often the family is there and sees that you are still rendering care and it is also a chance to check on the family. "You doin' OK?" It means a lot to them.

Rarely, I may feel the need to express my own opinion about what the patient would have wanted. Typically, this occurs when there is strong evidence that the patient will end as a Rankin 5 or 6, and that there is evidence from the family or friends that he would not want to survive as a Rankin 5 (and remember that 73% of Americans would not want that). Also, I become involved when the family cannot reach a judgement among themselves or if the majority of the family would withdraw life support measures but there is one very loud family member who will not agree. Often this family member has not been present at any of the GoC discussion in person, is angry about something (or has personal financial interests requiring the patient's survival) and is not going to be swayed by any line of reasoning. In that case, I will express my opinion something like this. "I rarely express an opinion in this matter but I am your father's doctor and, although I have been helping you up 'til now, my responsibility is to him first. He is my patient. All of the information points to the fact that either he is going to die no matter what we do or that he is going to end up severely disabled, requiring 24/7 nursing care in a nursing home. Everything you have told me about him leads me to believe that he would not want that. He hates doctors. He was a very independent person his whole life and was in a lot of pain before he was admitted. So I don't understand why you would force him to survive at this point. Wouldn't it be kinder to allow him to die peacefully when everything suggests that he would prefer that?"

There is an interesting dialogue that arises occasionally, it is not rare. A family member replies, "We want to let God's will be done and let Him take His course." I reply directly to this, with sympathy and understanding, but directly. "I'm afraid that is something that keeps me up at night. I can't know God's will. In fact, I often worry that I am standing in the way of God's will because, without our artificial machines and medical support, Mr. Harris would have died a week ago. So that just doesn't help us here." That is not likely to have an impact on the person who raised the point, although it might. But it is likely to be heard by everyone else in the family. By the way, I really do feel that way at times.

Organ donation is a whole world unto itself. We will consider it briefly in the chapter on ICU but for now I only want to make one brief but important point. It is well established that organ donation is much *less* likely to occur if it is raised initially by the treating team. You can appreciate the perceived conflict of interest. Therefore, it is essential that the treating team not be the ones to raise potential organ donation. This is referred to as "separation." This is one of the few hard "rules" that surrounds GoC. Frequently the family will raise the topic themselves and ask about organ donation. Your response should be simple and something like this. "Oh, that is really nice of you. Of course, we're not involved in that (motioning toward all of the staff in the room) but I can put you in touch with someone you can speak to. They'll be glad to spend time with you. Thank you." That's it, notify Gift of Life of the family's request and you're out.

Unnecessary Suffering

I'd like to tell you a story, two stories, actually.

I was receiving sign-out the night before coming on service in the Neuro ICU when the Attending signed out a "disastrous family member." The patient was severely injured by a prolonged cardiac arrest, was ventilator dependent, with complete loss of cerebral gray matter on MRI and flat line EEG but his wife was insistent that he receive tracheostomy and feeding tube for long term placement. There had been threatened law suits on both sides and no communication in more than a week. I actually received a call about the situation from our Chief Medical Officer later that night.

I can't tell you how unusual that is. Maybe once every five years this level of discord will occur. Maybe less. Anyway, Buddha says, "No matter how difficult the past, you can always begin again today." Changing Attendings is a good opportunity to try something new. So Monday morning I called his wife. There was no answer so I left a message. "Hi, this is Dr. Newman, I'll be taking care of your husband this week. Please call the ICU so we can speak." About an hour later she called and asked for me. I said "Hi!" again, she said "When will you do the trach." I said, "After I meet you. When can you come up?" After a brief pause, she agreed to meet the next day. The discussion that followed was unprecedented. I don't recommend it as a routine but circumstances were unique. Buddha also counsels us that when dealing with difficult people, we should "Imagine that each person in the world is enlightened but you. And that each person knows exactly the right thing to say and the right thing to do to teach you perfect patience, perfect wisdom and perfect compassion." It is never easy to learn this way but it happens. Something from every patient.

The lady presented on the unit the next morning with her teenage son. There was nothing visually outstanding about either. I brought them to a small conference room and she and I sat directly across from one another at a small table with her son at her side. Not really knowing how to proceed, for reasons that I cannot explain, out of the blue, I began by saying, "Before we start, I'd like us each to agree on one thing. I will agree that everything that you say and do, you say and do because you love him. I want you to agree that everything I say and do, I say and do because I want to avoid unnecessary suffering for your husband. I'll agree if you will." She sat back and looked me in the eyes for several long seconds. And then she responded, "OK."

We then proceeded to have a perfectly ordinary discussion, not much different than I would have with anyone else. In the end, I could not dissuade her from a course that all of the staff abhorred, but her relationship with staff became appropriate, almost cordial. He died, after having had the trach and PEG, almost immediately after transfer to a nursing home.

I don't ever remember using the term "unnecessary suffering" prior to that, in more than 40 years of practice. But I was amazed at how succinctly it summarized some very complex issues. That's the first story.

As often happens, a similar situation arouse shortly thereafter. In fact, the very next day I was asked by the medical ICU team to help a family member of another severely injured patient. The family member was having difficulty accepting the prognosis and wanted to proceed with trach and PEG even though the medical team believed further care to be futile. There was no animosity involved, it was a normal relationship.

Osler has two rules that we will discuss in the next chapter. "If it works, do it again. If it doesn't work, don't do it again." These are profound rules and I believe in them deeply. Anyway, "unnecessary suffering" had clearly worked once, so I purposefully intended to "do it again" with this family member. The family member asked to speak by phone. I don't like that but agreed. I reviewed the chart, saw the patient and we had a relatively routine discussion. He had clearly understood and digested the medical team's information. So after our discussion I said, simply, "You need to understand that your father's doctors really care about your father and they just want to avoid any unnecessary suffering on his part." The phone went silent. I don't know how long but it was long enough that I checked the phone display to ensure that we hadn't been disconnected. Then he said, "Doctor, you should bottle that. No one has ever said that to us. We have been wondering why they were advocating to allow him to die. Was it a matter of money? Did they need the bed? Are they hiding something? No one ever said anything like that to us. Thank you. I'll pick up again with the medical team. Good bye" And he hung up. But that's not the end of story.

I immediately went to speak with the MICU Attending to update her, of course. When I told her the same two stories that I just told you, she hit her forehead with her palm and said, "I have NEVER said that in any family meeting, but I will never have another family meeting where I don't say that."

Later that day, the son called the MICU Attending and let her know that the family agreed that withdrawal of life support measures and comfort care were what the patient would have wanted and they set up a time for palliative extubation.

We learn from our patients and sometimes from their families. Buddha knows.

Chapter 11. Some Principles of Clinical Pharmacology

Clinical pharmacology is a vast and rapidly changing field. Even introductory texts of pharmacology are large and complex. The goals of this chapter, on the other hand, are very simple. I would like to share four useful principles that have proven to be valuable guides throughout my career but that are often omitted from standard textbooks and courses. Two of these are gifts from Sir William Osler.

These four principles are:

1. How to add and subtract drugs from your drug armamentarium
2. The application of Osler's Rules to guide your medication experience
3. A simple, practical guide to dosing safety
4. Never let a potential side effect prevent you from using a drug that you need.

The first two principles are closely related.

Which Drugs Are You Going to Use?

When I was starting out as a medical student, a very senior Attending said to me, "The experienced physician is the last one to let a new drug in and the last one to let it out." He offered no explanation so I assumed that he meant for me to figure it out on my own and I have been trying to understand what he meant ever since.

I think that he meant that experienced physicians already have many drugs with which they are familiar and have already learned how to use those drugs optimally through long years of consistent practice. Therefore, that physician only lets in a new drug because they are aware of certain specific conditions for which they have no effective safe drug and are eager to try something new for that purpose. But then, when they finally encounter that situation and find a new drug which solves a particular problem, then they are hesitant to replace the drug with newer medications until they have established that the new medications are, in fact, more effective or safer than the old ones for that unique problem.

In other words, more senior physicians have developed substantial expertise using their preferred medications over decades of practice. It takes time to test new drugs in their practice so, in general, they are relatively conservative, slow to introduce newer drugs but also hesitant to relinquish drugs that they have found useful in a specific condition.

The exception to this conservative rule is a drug or other treatment that is introduced for a condition for which there is no known effective and safe treatment, especially if the new treatment is based on new knowledge emerging from basic and translational research. In that case, we are all eager to "give it a try."

Digoxin and phenobarbital are great examples of drugs "from antiquity" that remain on formulary. Many senior physicians still use digoxin to control heart rate in a fib either instead of or along with a beta-blocker such as metoprolol. Doesn't "dig" accumulate and produce yellow vision or even worsen atrial arrthymias? Isn't it hard to use if there is renal failure? The answer is "it can." But it is a potent positive inotrope and in uncompensated heart failure that may be very useful helping the patient tolerate higher doses of negative inotropes. So you will see an Attending hold the hand of a fellow or senior resident as they use dig, or phenobarbital in the case of refractory seizures, through their first episode. The fellow sees the benefit of the older drug under the experienced and cautious hand of their Attending and then they are ready to apply it themself the next time it is appropriate. We say, "See one, do one, teach one."

Let's explore further how a physician accumulates experience with new medications in a manner that is systematic and avoids excessive risk to their patients.

Osler's Rules

In the last chapter we applied one of Osler's Rules. Now I would like to introduce the two rules in a more general manner.

Rule #1. If it works, do it again.

Rule #2. If it doesn't work, don't do it again.

Uh, this probably needs some explanation; we expect a bit more from Osler.

Let's start with two obvious examples.

A patient with known multiple sclerosis presents with an exacerbation of left leg numbness that she has had previously. I wave a chicken over her head three times and 2 weeks later her symptoms have abated. Does that mean that waving a chicken over the person's head is a useful treatment for MS?

A second patient presents with glioblastoma multiforme. I treat that patient with cis-platinum and she dies 2 years later. Does that mean that cis-platinum is not useful for treating GBM?

The answer in both cases is obviously 'No.' Why?

Because the outcomes of both patients are within the expectation of the natural history (prognosis) of their diseases. Therefore, we cannot judge from those single experiences whether there was any effect on either patient.

Hmmm. Can we have more explanation? Sure! It seems that Osler must have had something more serious in mind for these rules.

First of all, there is the implication in these rules that you already have a sense of the natural history of the disease and that you are familiar with the range of responses of patients to the already available treatments.

Secondly, for some reason (see example below) you chose to avoid using the standard medications and, instead, used a medication that you never had used previously for this indication. When you did that, the question is whether the response of the patient exceeded the benefit that you had experienced with standard medications.

Let me give you a real example. The Stroke Team at the University of Wisconsin was taking care of a patient with crescendo TIAs. The patient was fluctuating rapidly between complete hemiplegia and a normal exam. This occurred several times within an hour right before our eyes. It is generally understood that these occur because of intermittent platelet plugging in diseased small penetrating arteries, in this case likely a lenticulostriate artery. The overwhelmingly likely result is the patient becomes hemiplegic despite available treatments. The CT scan was normal and his BP was not elevated. Dr. Doug Dulli was the stroke attending. All stroke team members were at bedside discussing how to get aspirin and Plavix into this patient as quickly as possibly when Dr. Dulli cut us off and said, "To hell with this, I'm going to start abciximab", a potent and immediate IV antiplatelet agent. None of us had ever done that or read about its use for that purpose but we all agreed and the drug was given stat. There were no further TIAs. Oral antiplatelets were started the next day and the patient left the hospital, completely intact, Rankin 0, a day later. Yeah!

What did we take away from this? Did we "know" that abciximab had worked? No, the outcome is not uniformly disastrous so it was possible that the attack simply ended spontaneously. But all of us were struck with the temporal relationship and the sense that this was way outside of the usual course. Based on Osler's Rule #1, we felt that "it worked." Our response as modern physicians, was to formulate the hypothesis that abciximab may be able to improve the outcome in crescendo TIAs. Crescendo TIAs are not common but they are not rare and their outcome is often a life changing event for the patient. We agreed as a team that we would use abciximab in the future when a patient presented with crescendo TIAs. Since it had worked, we would do it again; cautiously. Over the next two years, we treated 8 additional patients with rapidly fluctuating neurologic deficits consistent with crescendo TIAs, administering the abciximab while they were neurologically intact with normal CT, and not one of them went on to complete their stroke or have a bleeding complication. That is completely outside of statistical likelihood to be by chance alone.

Let's reflect on this a bit. Abciximab is not without risk, especially in acute stroke. Our reasoning was that tissue infarction had not yet occurred since he had a normal neurologic exam when we gave the drug. So the risk seemed reasonable in the face of a highly probable outcome of hemiplegia. We observed the patient very carefully and maintained tight control over his BP to mitigate risk of bleeding or hypotension. We withheld all other blood thinning medications for the same reason. Why not try anticoagulation or intensive oral anti-platelet? Because all of us had experience that those drugs had not been effective when we used them for crescendo TIAs in the past.

But what about Rule #2? Well, there are plenty of examples of this. I had a patient with NMDA encephalitis who was in status epilepticus controlled only by pentobarbital for a total of 3 months despite conventional anti-epileptic drugs. Several people recommended that I try ketamine. Nothing else was working and the risk seemed reasonable so I did. Her EEG changed in interesting ways, but as soon as I took away the pentobarb with IV ketamine plus her seizure meds, the seizures returned. She eventually did well with immunomodulation, as is often the case, but I haven't tried ketamine again in NMDA encephalitis since then. I have also tried ketamine once as a neuroprotectant after a paper demonstrated consistently poor outcome in cardiac arrest patients who experience myoclonic seizures with usual management. It didn't improve the outcome in that patient either. Maybe if I tried more. Maybe, but I didn't. Formal research might prove otherwise. I look forward to reading the paper.

I want to give you another example of Rule #2 by continuing the stroke story from Rule #1. During the series of 8 additional patients, the hospital administration came to me in my role as Stroke Director and asked if we could use Integrilin instead of abciximab because the mechanisms are similar and the drug is much cheaper. They added immediately that they did not want me to jeopardize anyone's outcome and that I should use it only if I thought the results would be equivalent. I told them I didn't know but, given the potential severity of the condition, I wasn't really comfortable making the switch. They accepted that and we kept using abciximab.

Now I'm an opportunist. By that I mean, there are many trials of patient care that I would love to try but cannot justify because I am not at equipoise and feel there would be uncertain patient risk. But sometimes, the experiment that you would like to do is the only option and it becomes acceptable or actually necessary. That is the sense that I mean when I say I am an opportunist. This is a useful corollary for Osler's Rules.

So, to continue our crescendo TIA story, the UW Stroke Program routinely maintained close affiliations with most neurologists throughout the state. One day a friend from a mid-sized hospital called and wanted my advice for a patient having crescendo TIAs. I told him about our experience with abciximab and recommended that he try it. He paused and then said, we don't use abciximab here, it's not on formulary. Can I try Integrilin? Opportunity knocks! Now we had to do the experiment that we had wanted to do but were not comfortable doing. So we tried the integrilin since it was the only drug available. Unfortunately, it did not stop the crescendo TIAs and the patient completed his stroke. Was that proof that Integrilin wouldn't work? No. But we never considered using Integrilin instead of abciximab again.

Let's step back and digest all of this. There are several points related to Osler's rules. First, we must be familiar with the natural history of the diseases we treat as well as the expected benefit of the standard drugs used for each condition. Secondly, by being consistent in our use of medication, consistently using one medication at a time for a specific indication in order to understand its value and its failings, we gradually learn the spectrum of conditions for which the drug will and will not work. If we are not consistent or do not observe the outcomes carefully, then we will not learn and will not improve our patient care. When we encounter a specific condition for which the drugs that we usually use are not effective, then we begin to seek alternative agents and are justified in accepting more risk than usual if the risk of disease progression outweighs the likely drug complications. If the outcome of a "trial" with one patient is better than our expectation based on prior experience, then we consider using the drug again the next time we encounter that condition. If, however, the result is no better than the standard drugs, then we try something else next time. In essence, we learn how to improve our treatments one patient at a time. That is, we learn from our patients. Where have I heard that before?

Calculate the Dose, Give Half, Observe, Give the Other Half (Maybe)

You will encounter many situations where you will calculate the dose of some medication based on weight or estimated measured metabolic deficit. The drug could be digoxin, or sodium or free water replacement, or first dose of furosemide, or valproic acid. Now for some drugs, such as antibiotics, anti-rejection drugs and many chemotherapeutic agents, you just go ahead and give the calculated dose, which is often adjusted for age, weight, renal and liver function. But for many physiologically active drugs, especially those affecting the heart, cardiovascular system and nervous system, a useful guideline is to give half of the calculated dose, observe the effect on the patient and then give more. "More" may be the second half or it might be less than half depending on the magnitude of the response to the first half. I could give countless examples where I was glad that I had followed this rule.

The thing is, you can always put in more but it's very hard to take out what you have put in. Always consider whether you want to follow this rule in any particular case. If the drug is physiologically active and has affects which can be observed at the bedside, including blood pressure, heart rate, ventilation or urine output, then consider taking this approach.

A corollary of this is expressed in the analogy of "tiptoeing away from the edge" when someone is critically ill. For some reason, when I approach a patient on the verge of catastrophe, I see them in my mind as if they are standing at a deep precipice, with their toes on the edge of a steep abyss, and leaning forward as if about to fall in. I visualize my initial goal as simply to put my hands on their shoulders and get them to lean back toward me, away from the abyss. Then I want to slowly walk them backwards, "tiptoeing away from the edge." My concern is that if I grab their shoulders and pull hard, their feet might slip and I will be left hanging onto them after they have fallen into the abyss. I don't like that image at all. I've seen too many movies where that happens and they lose their grip so that the patient falls and dies.

What am I saying? I'm saying that while it is often necessary to take quick and decisive action in a critical situation, it is possible to be overly aggressive and create new problems with our treatments. It is essential to act quickly and hold onto the patient but a hard jerk isn't always the correct action. Sometimes a firm and steady pull is better.

Dosing considerations also lead naturally to a discussion of infusions. You will nearly always get a steadier serum level with an infusion than with frequent boluses. For one thing, nurses will make very small and frequent adjustments to the rate of an infusion but they are much less inclined to give frequent boluses. There's more work involved with a bolus than simply changing the rate on a pump. I've always believed that there is some psychological reason as well but maybe not since I never identified one.

Infusion has one significant disadvantage, however, and that is slower onset of action, depending on the first elimination half-life of the drug and the rate of infusion. Also, very small volume infusions take a long time to clear through the IV tubing, which may be 2 to 4 ml in volume, before hitting the blood stream. As a result, the ideal delivery method is often a "loading" bolus followed by infusion. This usually permits a rapid onset and sustained action with lower risk than a large bolus which can produce a high transient peak and initial toxicity. Fentanyl, pentobarbital and lidocaine are good examples of this bolus-infusion technique but there are many, many others.

Never Let a Potential Complication Prevent You from Using a Drug that the Patient Needs.

This is another recommendation that is often attributed to Osler. On reading it, your response might well be "Duh, no kidding." However, I will tell you that I often find the need to cite this recommendation in order to overcome the inhibition of junior or even senior physicians who are thinking *primum non nocere*, "first do no harm."

Read Osler's recommendation carefully. This is a drug that the patient NEEDS. The side effect is POTENTIAL. Consider a common Neuro ICU example.

The patient was originally admitted with a right hemispheric intracerebral hematoma five days ago. Today he developed shortness of breath and was found to have segmental pulmonary emboli with DVT in his plegic left leg. From this point on, specifics would matter but let's assume that he was hemodynamically stable enough that IR didn't feel that thrombectomy is warranted. The MICU team believed strongly that he should be started on heparin.

What should his Neuro ICU team do? Most of us would say that starting heparin is a no brainer. Why? He needs it! The PE is life threatening. His ICH was 5 days ago and he may well tolerate the heparin without further bleeding. But I would also say that the last thing in the world I would want for this patient is a supratherapeutic PTT. Therefore, I calculate the heparin dose, almost certainly omit a bolus, and start the infusion at about 60% of the calculated infusion rate to avoid the potential overdose. Doesn't that increase the risk that the PE will worsen? Yes, a little, but I am "balancing risks" or "hedging my bet" whichever way you choose to express it. And I speak to the nurse <u>before</u> every scheduled change in infusion rate to ensure that the recommendation of the hospital's heparin nomogram is applicable to my patient. I write that as an order in the chart. There's much less tolerance for variability in this case. To emphasize this, I often say to the team "There's no room for sloppiness here, we need to pull our belts tight!"

Buddha says, "Blessings come from care, troubles from carelessness."

I don't let the potential complication prevent me from using a drug that the patient needs but I am obsessively compulsive in monitoring my patient given the risks.

¿Tiene sentido?

Chapter 12. Introduction to the ICU

Just as with Pharmacology, this is a tremendously complex subject and there are many excellent references available. This chapter is not intended to substitute for them, it is merely a collection of ideas that I have found useful for introducing students and residents to intensive care. The purpose is to help you acclimate easily to the ICU which can be intimidating initially because of its unique features as a place of practice.

Secondary Prevention in the ICU

I gradually developed the understanding that a central purpose of an ICU is secondary prevention. In most cases, the disease that landed them in the ICU has already been addressed in the field, the ED, the OR or other units of the hospital. They survived and were stabilized enough to move them to the ICU. The next phase is not only to continue the primary management, but also to avoid or mitigate new complications of the primary problem and its treatment.

There was a paper in the New England Journal in 2009 that made me focus on the idea of secondary prevention. The original hypothesis was that the best surgical hospitals in the US would have fewer complications than the worst surgical hospitals. Duuuuuuh! Obvious, right? But no, that hypothesis turned out to be false! Fewer complications did not explain the better results in the top rated hospitals. Huh? Then what does? It is the speed with which the best hospitals respond to the complications. Ahhhh! So, it seems that the best hospitals anticipate the complications that they know are likely to occur. They put in place reliable monitoring programs and have plans already prepared if the patient does develop the problem along with specific thresholds for taking action. This paper completely changed my approach to the ICU.

Variation in Hospital Mortality Associated with Inpatient Surgery
Ghaferi, AA, Birkmeyer JD, and Dimick JB. N Engl J Med 2009;361:1368-1375
DOI: 10.1056/NEJMsa0903048

From that point on, I viewed the ICU as a place to continue the initial management as well as to manage or prevent the numerous severe complications that are common in critically ill patients. In a certain sense, patient management in the ICU involves "looking for trouble." This conceptual approach alters everything, from patient rounds to statistical judgements.

An organ system approach is standard for keeping track of patient management in the ICU. Every organ needs to be considered. But "looking for trouble" focuses us not just on what is but on what might be. It is not just a matter of knowing how well the organ is functioning and what management is in place to maintain or improve the function. It is also necessary to ask whether each organ is at risk to develop new problems given the patient's existing problems and management. Some of this is obvious. Delayed cerebral ischemia is a recognized complication of subarachnoid hemorrhage. But there are many more subtle, less common potential complications that also should be monitored.

This approach can create discomfort among physicians who do not think this way. For instance, as a consultant, I might see a potentially serious complication with a 2% likelihood of occurring in a particular patient. I might see a relatively simple management plan that would reduce that risk and provide an early alert if the complication becomes more likely. But when I discuss this with the ICU Attending, the plan may be rejected because it is so unlikely. Unfortunately, if we treat 50 such patients, one will suffer the catastrophic complication that might have been prevented.

Let's be careful here. It is incumbent upon me to ensure that the "cost" of my preventive management is low enough and the consequences of the rare event are high enough (death, severe disability or prolonged hospital stay) to justify implementing the strategy in the face of the low probability. But there are plenty of times when those conditions are easily met. Often a simple monitoring tool based on focused physical exam or vital signs is all that is necessary. We have already discussed the need for meticulous BP management in a patient with ICH being heparinized for a PE. Sometimes just communicating with the anesthesiologist prior to a procedure is sufficient. Neither action is expensive or risky.

Talking to the ICU Nurse

By way of introduction and to get the attention of new students and residents, I often say "If you walk into an ICU room without first talking to the patient's nurse, then you are a fool." Hyperbole aside, I mean that the ICU nurse is the only one who really knows exactly what is going on with the patient. Virtually nothing can happen without the nurse and good ICU nurses are completely up to date on every aspect of their patient's status. It's true that ICU nurses take care of two patients and something may change while they are with the other patient or that plans have been made but not yet discussed with the nurse, but that doesn't change my recommendation. It's also possible that there have been changes in the patient's status or plans which have not yet been charted by anyone. Therefore, I strongly recommend that you talk to the ICU nurse before entering the patient's room. That also helps to develop the cordial working relationship that you want and makes the nurse aware of your visit so that it gets charted. "Dr. Newman in to see patient at 0850." That can be very useful for many purposes.

Also, before I enter the room, I am certain to speak with a member of my team, or the primary ICU team if I am a consultant. I like to pull the primary team's junior resident aside for a brief conversation while the ICU team is making bedside rounds. I also will have reviewed the most recent primary care team's progress notes and any recent notes from new or ongoing consultants such as renal, ID, endocrinology, hematology, hepatology or others, before entering the room. I will also review new labs, imaging and electrophysiology before seeing the patient.

Upon Entering the Patient's Room

I am not suggesting what follows as "the right way." This is just how

I do it.

On entering the room of an ICU patient, I first note if there are any visitors. If there are, and we have already met, then I greet them, without shaking hands, and make simple pleasantry. If we have not previously met then I introduce myself. "Hi! I'm Dr. George Newman, one of the neurologists in the ICU." I wait for them to introduce themselves. I need to know how they are related to the patient in order to know how much information I should share with them. If their relationship is remote, I may ask them to wait outside the room "while I examine the patient and speak with his nurse."

Visitors aside, I have a simple routine on entering an ICU room. Understand that I am with the patient's nurse so that I can share my thoughts and ask questions continuously throughout the visit. I look at the patient for a preliminary survey, then I look at the monitor, then I look at the ventilator, then I look at the IV medication pumps. I make sure to ask the nurse about recent events or management changes, when they occurred, and imminent plans for testing or procedures. Then I return to the patient for a more thorough evaluation.

My preliminary patient survey is to screen for obvious signs of shock, determine ventilatory status and review what tubes and lines are in place. What is the apparent level of consciousness? Are there overt seizures or grossly abnormal limb postures? I am also very conscious of odors in the room, they are important clues to infections and metabolic problems.

From the monitor, I learn the BP, heart rate and rhythm, whether an arterial line is in use, whether there are intracranial or other special monitors, and the oxygen saturation (SaO_2).

From the ventilator settings I see the ventilator mode (such as control, assist, pressure support or CPAP), the FiO_2 being delivered, the set respiratory rate and the patient's rate, the peek pressure, the presence of PEEP and the shape of the pressure curves. From the combination of FiO_2 and SaO_2 I form a rough estimate of gas exchange and from the peak pressure curve I get a rough estimate of airway resistance.

From the medication pumps, I can see the current level of sedation through the combination of anesthetics and pain medications, the pressor support or antihypertensives being used as well as any anti-arrhythmic agents. Antibiotics and anti-seizure medications are more intermittent so that I have to ask about those while I am discussing the specific reasons for each running med with the nurse.

All of this information is then combined with the information from the nurse, my chart review and conversation with other team members in order to form an overall impression of the current status of the patient. Most importantly, are they improving, stable or worsening, and which, if any, organs are failing. I then ask myself what role I need to play for this patient. Perhaps none. At one extreme, I may simply do a reality check that I am not needed with the nurse and leave. At the other extreme, I may perceive the need for immediate action and get a member of my team or the primary team to join me to act in concert. In the large majority of cases, however, I simply proceed to a more thorough examination.

One word of caution. Be careful to avoid inadvertently pulling out lines, extubating the patient or tripping on equipment. You lose a lot of points if you do any of those. An ICU room is often crowded with equipment that is connected to the patient in one way or another. When you move in the room, look carefully at the floor to be sure that there are no lines or tubing in your path. When you approach the bedside, choose a "path" which gets you to the patient with the least physical interference and as you examine the patient, be careful to avoid movements of the head or limbs that risk dislodging critical connectors, especially the ET or trach tube. Believe me, it happens. Fortunately, the nurse doesn't trust anyone around the bedside so that they are usually monitoring your movements and are ready to intervene to avoid such occurrences.

There are many patients in the ICU who are alert and cooperative. In those patients, the usual neurologic history and exam applies. The neurologic exam of patients in coma is a simplified version of the usual neurologic exam with the addition of several reflexes, especially involving the eyes. As with the formal neurologic exam, I prefer to refer you to any of the excellent available texts. Instead I want to focus here on lessons that I have learned that are not usually emphasized in those books. Let's start with how to assess and report the level of consciousness.

Assessing and Reporting Level of Consciousness (LOC)

I usually begin with my students by explaining that I know what alert means and I know what comatose means but all other words that describe LOC are ambiguous. A simple example suffices. You are on call at night and the ICU nurse calls and asks you to evaluate a patient because he seems less responsive than earlier in the day. You examine the patient and then look at the progress note from the day team where the patient is described as "lethargic." There is no way for you to determine whether the patient is better, worse or unchanged. Therefore I recommend a simple operational description that avoids this predicament.

First of all, "alert" means that the patient is actively perceiving their environment and anticipating what is to come. To explain, you walk into a bar alert but when you walk out after a few drinks you are much less attentive and vigilant than earlier. You are no longer alert, which is why you shouldn't drive. Secondly, "comatose" means that the person does not respond with any degree of arousal to any stimuli. Thus, "alert" and "comatose" can be defined reasonably precisely. So far so good. Now let's deal with everything in between.

Basically, LOC can be described by three factors related to the patient's best response.

1. What stimulus was used to elicit the best response?
2. What was the best response?
3. How long did the best response persist without further

stimulation?

A couple of examples might help, then we'll look more systematically at these factors.

Example #1
I walk into our apartment and you are on the couch sleeping. I call your name and then tap you on the shoulder gently. You wake up with a start, rub your face and eyes, and then are ready to go study (or party).
1. Stimulus was gentle voice and gentle tactile stimulation (stim).
2. Best response was fully alert.
3. Duration was for the duration of the rest of my exam.

Example #2
I walk into the ICU and examine a patient with eyes closed. I call his name repeatedly and loudly, tap and then shake his shoulder. Finally I pinch the skin of his shoulder quite hard. He mumbles a few unintelligible words without opening his eyes and returns to his earlier state within seconds.
1. Stimuli were loud voice, vigorous tactile and light noxious.
2. Best response was vocalization without verbalization, without eye opening
3. Duration was several seconds.

With this type of simple procedure for examining and reporting the LOC, anyone can review your note from earlier, repeat a similar exam and accurately compare the patient's current and prior exams. And the nurse will get the answer they need.

Typical stimuli for this exam include "spontaneously" (that is no stimuli were needed). "Spontaneous" is exactly that. I walk into the room and the patient is sitting up doing something or interacting with someone, no stimulation at all is needed to observe their LOC. Note that they might not be alert though, they may only be awake or aroused but not alert. That's a different matter to be discussed momentarily.

Let me make clear right now that I am not a fan of noxious stimulation. The initial exam and some subsequent exams may require noxious stim for LOC but I regularly see noxious stim overutilized in the ICU. If the patient's limb is lying flaccid as part of an obvious hemiplegia, does it make sense for me to apply intense noxious stim to see if I can elicit a reflex or some other response? I would say that the information gained is not worth the potential pain, the lack of humane treatment and the possible conditioning of the patient to the approach of other care givers. Even when noxious stim is indicated for LOC, I would prefer to ask the nurse what was found and not repeat that part of the exam if possible. I have also learned to correlate abnormal limb postures and flaccid tone with lack of response to noxious stimuli and so can frequently avoid it.

Anyway, with those stimuli, we might observe a variety of responses such as fully alert, or awake but not alert; fully cooperative, or intermittently cooperative, or minimally cooperative with repeated stim; or verbal, or vocalizing without verbalizing, or moaning; or eye opening with fixation, or eye opening without fixation; or localizing stimuli, or arousing without localizing, or minimal generalized response, or no response. Note that you can combine ocular, vocal and motor descriptions for the response. You might also note the relation to the Glasgow Coma Scale. It is a good idea to calculate and report the GCS as well since that number can be followed over time and is very well standardized. The difference of this approach from the GCS, however, is that these responses are closely associated with a specified stimulus and duration of the response.

People can be awake but not alert even if their eyes are open, they listen to and perform instructions, and speak intelligibly. But they may form little memory, miss interpersonal cues, and fail to recognize your behavioral patterns or plans. For example, if I tap the DTR of your right arm, you probably would expect me to tap the left arm as well and you probably would help me reach your left arm. You are alert and cooperative, as well as very nice. But many ICU patients who appear awake don't do that. They are missing cues, not generalizing, not anticipating, not participating. They are passive and inattentive. They are awake but not alert.

Obviously, you will need the help of the family or of doctors, nurse or therapists who knew the patient before the present episode in order to know how far their current status is from their recent baseline. The chart may contain that information, or not. It is amazing to me how often the family of a patient with prior head trauma or other brain injury will say, "Oh, yeah. That's pretty good for him." No need for further work-up.

How long they maintain that best response is obvious. How many seconds or minutes or was it "for the remainder of the exam?"

Now we need to understand WHY the patient's LOC is what it is. More exam and more hypotheses to be tested.

Why Is This Patient Not Awake?

Remember that Neurology, including Neurocritical Care, is applied neuroanatomy. So a basic question is, what are the neuroanatomic structures which can result to altered consciousness when they fail? Most correctly point to the reticular activating system (RAS) as one source. The second less obvious cause is failure of both cerebral hemispheres diffusely. Truthfully, lesser degrees of altered consciousness can come from numerous structures, especially the thalamus and the insula, but in the ICU, the useful clinical guideline is that altered consciousness reflects failure of either the RAS or the cerebral hemispheres diffusely.

A fundamental clinical question in patients with altered LOC is, therefore, whether there is a structural anatomic lesion involving the RAS or not.

The RAS extends longitudinally in the midline of the brainstem from the medulla into the thalamus but, with rare exceptions, it works well to think of it as near the midline of the upper pons and midbrain. Because pathways for pupillary reactivity and eye movements are in these same anatomic regions of the brainstem and are relatively resistant to systemic insults such as systemic organ failure, sepsis or drug toxicities, the examination of coma and altered LOC relies heavily on examination of the eyes. Of course, the basic guideline that asymmetry or focal findings strongly suggests a structural lesion applies equally well in coma as in any other neurologic problem. But a focal lesion, in an of itself, is unlikely to be the cause of a major change in LOC unless it involves the RAS.

When there is no evidence of a structural brainstem lesion in a patient with significantly impaired LOC, then it is reasonable to assume that the patient has bilateral hemisphere dysfunction. This is usually referred to as an encephalopathy. When I encounter a probable encephalopathy, I always remind myself of the clinical correlates of encephalopathy with a simple sing-song. "Toxic, metabolic, infectious, and sometimes post-ictal." These considerations should guide your evaluations. However, diffusely increased ICP, from severe hydrocephalus or hepatic failure, can also present this way. And watch out for thalamic lesions.

Principles of the Doll's Eye Maneuver (Oculocephalic Reflex)

In this brief section, I would like to present the principles of the oculocephalic maneuver, commonly referred to as Doll's Eyes, because it is one of the most useful signs in the ICU and is often misinterpreted. I like the term doll's eyes because understanding how a real baby doll's eyes work is useful to understand the sign and how we describe the findings.

The concept of doll's eyes is derived directly from the baby doll's function which is illustrated in the figure below. Basically, a baby doll is awake with eyes open when the doll is vertical but is asleep with eyes closed when the doll is horizontal. As can be seen in this simple drawing, it is the head that moves. **The eyes remain fixed in**

space. That is the key. When the head moves, the eyes do not.

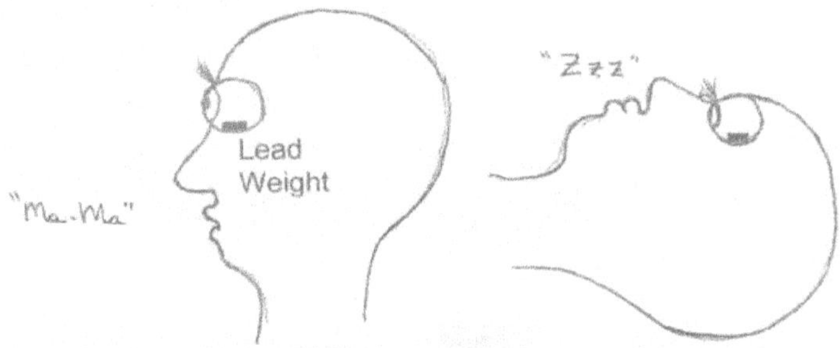

The oculocephalic, or doll's eyes, maneuver is performed by rotating the head laterally to both side, not vertically, but the principle is identical. In a patient "with doll's eyes," when the head is rotated, the eyes remain fixed in space. Assuming that the eyes were in primary position before the maneuver, the eyes continue to look toward the ceiling during the movement. Some movement at the end of the maneuver can be ignored.

What does it mean if doll's eyes are present? It means that the oculocephalic reflex is intact. Let's assume the head is turned to the right. Briefly, the oculocephalic reflex involves vestibular input from the right semicircular canal through right CN VIII and the output involves the right CN VI for abducting the right eye and left CN III for adducting the left eye. The brainstem nuclei for CN VIII and CN VI are in the mid to lower pons on the right but left CN III is at the top of the midbrain contralaterally. The connection is via the medial longitudinal fascicular (MLF) which traverses the pons and midbrain close to the midline. That means that the MLF is running right through the RAS which occupies the same position.

So here's the punch line. If doll's eyes are present, then you know two things unambiguously. The first is that the patient really does have altered consciousness. People who are awake do not have doll's eyes, their eyes will "follow their nose" and not remain fixed in space. This helps identify patients in the ICU with reduced LOC and helps identify fictitious coma in the ED. The second thing you know, however, is that the cause of the patient's altered LOC is not a structural lesion in the brainstem. This is precisely the information that we needed. It is, therefore, very likely that the patient has dysfunction of both cerebral hemispheres diffusely, that is that they have an encephalopathy. That distinction is what makes this test one of the most valuable physical signs in the ICU.

If the oculocephalic reflex produces a partial response then it is very likely that there is a brainstem lesion. If there is no response and the eyes remain fixed in the orbit, then either there is a severe brainstem lesion or a profound depression of global brain function, or the patient is actually awake and this is fictitious coma. Thus, the absence of doll's eyes requires further investigation for interpretation. It is the presence of doll's eyes that is immediately useful.

Treating Comatose Patients with Respect

Sometimes it is difficult to see the comatose patient in the ICU as a person because we are deeply involved in sorting through the myriad problems involved in management. In addition, the reality is that there are many factors which disturb our own senses and sensibilities when patients are critically ill. Infections smell. Patients defecate at any given moment. Wounds may extrude pus which is putrid by sight and smell. That's a basic aspect of the ICU but it can lead to a dehumanization of the patient.

My first response in this setting is to acknowledge these features to the nurse and commiserate with his or her constant contact with these aspects of the patient. I also will sympathize with family, again by acknowledging and providing hope that these are unavoidable but temporary aspects of the patient's hospitalization. Then I deal with myself. I literally step back and warn myself. First, I need to exert extra caution to avoid contaminating my person which brings risk to myself, my family and my next patient. Then I need to remind myself that this is a person who deserves my compassion, my respect and my best efforts for their medical care.

I want to reiterate my aversion to producing pain in patients with altered LOC. They may be sensitive to pain even when not awake. Some patients will even be awake or nearly so but "locked in" without the motor responses to indicate their near conscious state. It frightens and saddens me to think how often I have seen noxious stimuli used in a patient that I consider at least partially responsive. The same thing applies to the spoken word. I am always concerned about the possibility that a patient may intermittently be alert enough to hear and understand our bedside comments. For that reason, I always avoid pejorative speech or statements of apocalyptic prognosis at the bedside. In fact, if I have any sense that the patient is improving or intermittently arousing, I usually ask the nurse to place a large note at the head of the bed indicating this and warning others to avoid noxious stimuli or careless speech.

One final comment concerns how you relate, physically, to the patient while speaking with the family in the patient's room. The goal is to convey your compassion and respect non-verbally as you provide the verbal medical update. Somewhat surprisingly, many of us who work in the ICU have independently worked out a common strategy to achieve this which has to do with where we stand when we speak with the family. Basically, we stand on the side of the bed opposite from the family and look across the patient while speaking to the family members. At the same time, we place our hand on the patient in a manner that would suggest comforting, sometimes just a touch, sometimes a subtle caress. When providing emphasis to a point verbally to the family, we might tap the patient gently as a means of involving them. Never mind if the patient has been comatose for a week, we still follow this simple approach. It achieves the goal of letting the family know that we consider their loved one a person with feelings without having to say so. Any verbal expression of the same would be extremely awkward but becomes unnecessary by doing this.

Death in the ICU

Critically ill patients are at high risk for dying. That is the reality.

Death is an intrinsic part of the ICU. This is something that you must learn to manage in yourself as well as others. I would not say that you ever get used to it, I hope you don't. I never have. But you have to learn to manage the intense feelings of the family and, sometimes, in the staff and yourself. It is natural to have more intense feelings with younger patients, in those occupying a central role in the family, with more sudden illnesses or injuries and in those with whom you have had a prior relationship. It's not that anyone is "more important" than anyone else. It's just our nature, there is no point in denying it.

To this day, I remember my very first patient in the hospital when I was a third year medical student. The patient was actually very stable but had moderate respiratory distress from congestive heart failure. As I interviewed him, I kept thinking, "Please don't die while I'm in here with you." The idea of experiencing the death of a patient was very disturbing. But I also remember mid-way through my internship that a young woman with Eisenmenger's physiology and hemoptysis was admitted to my service one night. I was told without equivocation by her Attending that she was going to die while on my service. I remember spending the night with her, at times holding her to comfort her as she was still conscious and knew she was dying. She died in my arms before sunrise. I was no longer afraid, my compassion had overcome my fear. That night remains an emotional memory even now as I write about it, but I never feared death again. It is likely that you will have similar experiences. You can't prepare, not really. You can only respond and do your best to provide comfort when the moment arrives.

Chapter 13. Brain Death

Why Do We Need Brain Death Protocols?

When the positive pressure ventilator and ICU's were invented, it became possible to sustain people who had suffered severe irreversible brain injury indefinitely even though they remained permanently comatose. Autopsies revealed that their brains had autolyzed to liquid encephalomalacia. This was unacceptable to everyone involved. Therefore the states (in the United States) created laws that permitted determination of death by cessation of brain function, commonly referred to as Brain Death.

Here is the entire Pennsylvania statute.

> "Pennsylvania Statutes Title 35 P.S. Health and Safety § 10203.
> Determination of death
> Current as of January 01, 2022
>
> Only an individual who has sustained either:
> (1) irreversible cessation of circulatory and respiratory functions; or
> (2) irreversible cessation of all functions of the entire brain, including the brain stem is dead.
>
> A determination of death must be made in accordance with accepted medical standards."

It is incumbent upon every medical center to maintain a protocol to ensure that determination of death is in accord with accepted medical standards. This is a topic of active debate and research around the world right now. As usual, I will opt for a simple approach based on my own experience.

Before such laws, crazy things happened. My first year on the faculty at Stony Brook in 1981 I declared a patient dead using standardized criteria after the patient was shot in the head and had herniated.

However, 6 months later, the defendant's defense was that I had killed the patient, not the shooter. Fortunately, the jury took only 10 minutes to decide that wasn't true, but it helps illustrate why there was need for laws.

My first Chair, Dr. Robert Y Moore served on an early Federal committee to recommend brain death guidelines. When he returned from Washington he said they had decided that brain death could be defined as "areflexic, apneic, coma." The patient was not responsive to any stimuli, there were no brain reflexes present, and the patient did not breathe spontaneously. What was needed was to provide operational definitions of how to establish these three features.

Brain Death Determination

There are multiple protocols available online and I encourage anyone interested to review one or more. The following discussion is based on the protocol at Einstein - Jefferson Medical Center in 2023. The protocol is intended to run with minimal medical decisions, with each step fully specified and with very few options, each of which has completely specified criteria. Reporting is rigidly standardized.

What triggers the brain death protocol? Anytime any member of the treatment team suggests out loud that they do not see any evidence of brain function, then that automatically triggers the protocol. Einstein continues to use two bedside examinations at least 6 hours apart plus a formal apnea test. Many medical centers now use a single bedside exam. We retained two not for scientific reasons but to help our community accept the finality. Two different ways of performing the apnea test are permitted in case of cardiovascular instability. A "confirmatory test" was used only if some other part of the protocol was not possible for a clinical reason such as bandaged eyes or unstable cardiovascular status that prohibited either apnea test.

There is more to the protocol than just the determination itself. For instance, the Einstein protocol begins by educating the family about brain death. That is the first step so that they are aware and can follow the process throughout. That helps them accept the finality of the determination. The protocol specifies who may perform the examinations. The two exams must be done by two different doctors. The protocol also specifies approximately the time frame over which the determination occurs as well as how long the family may have with the patient after the patient is declared dead. Without these aspects being specified, family members can introduce delays that may be unacceptable to other family members as well as the health care team and medical center.

The exam for Brain Death is similar to the usual examination of coma but makes greater use of cold water calorics and deep noxious stimuli. There also are criteria intended to eliminate factors which may mimic brain death including certain types of drugs, severe metabolic disturbances, hypotension, hypothermia and hypoxia.

The exam criteria are relatively simple and recorded in two categories.

Loss of Cerebral Function
1. Response to painful stimuli is absent
2. Muscular movements except spinal reflexes are absent

Loss of Brain Stem Function
1. Pupils are fixed
2. Corneal reflexes are absent
3. Oculocephalic reflexes are absent (no eye movement to Dolls' Eyes maneuver)
4. Oculovestibular reflexes are absent (no eye movement to 50ml of ice water in
   each ear canal)
5. Gag response and cough to tracheal stimulation are absent

That's all there is. If there is evidence of complete loss of cerebral and brain stem function on two separate exams 6 hours apart as well as absence of respiratory effort on a formal exam, then the patient is declared legally dead at the time of the second exam or apnea test, the later of the two.

The purpose of a "confirmatory test" is to demonstrate the absence of blood flow. By protocol this may be done by nuclear medicine flow study or conventional angiography. In practice, the nuclear medicine study is always used. The absence of cerebral blood flow is demonstrated by the "hot nose" finding where radioactive tracer to the nose stands out against a dark background due to the absence of perfusion inside the cranium.

The medical aspects really are as simple as they seem. The harder part is helping the family understand and accept this process. This takes place in one or more family meetings. In truth, the meeting is much simpler than a GoC discussion described earlier because it is mainly an informational meeting about the protocol. The extreme complexity of the GoC discussion is completely absent. Yet, like everything else in medicine, there are skills to be learned that help reach the goal more effectively and with less family distress.

Meeting with the Family

The family and staff are assembled in the same manner as for GoC. There is usually one presenter for the staff, often a neurologist but can be neurosurgeon or intensivist. The presenter should be experienced in the protocol and have participated in numerous meetings before taking the lead role.

I think it is important to maintain a fairly matter of fact attitude for this type of meeting. Obviously we need to show compassion but we need to convey that this is going to happen, how it will happen, how we will communicate and how we will act depending on our findings on the various exams. In a sense, we have become part of the protocol.

When I am the leader, I begin simply by thanking them for coming and then say that there has been a change in status of their father and that we need to discuss that with them. I continue by saying that one of the doctors or nurses (whichever it was) has raised a concern that they do not see "evidence of brain function." That is a specific phrase I will use repeatedly. I then continue, "whenever that happens, it automatically triggers a brain death protocol, and that is what we need to discuss." I then explain briefly to them why brain death laws were created and that state law requires us to have a protocol to establish whether there is or is not evidence of brain function because if there is no evidence of brain function then he will be declared dead." I go on to emphasize that there are no decisions in this protocol, not by them and not by me. "The protocol runs like a train on a track. It has to because otherwise this is too difficult."

I continue by explaining the protocol in some detail, similar to the above. I emphasize that none of us would ever want to make a mistake in such matters so that at least two different doctors are involved, usually three including the apnea test. I explain that the purpose is to see if there is brain function so that, after each exam the examiner will come out and say either that they do or that they do not see evidence of brain function. I go step by step. "If the first exam does not show evidence of brain function then the protocol will continue but if there is ANY evidence of brain function, then the protocol ends and your father will not be declared dead." I repeat that for the apnea test and then repeat it a third time for the second bedside exam. I emphasize that on the apnea test his breathing does not have to be effective, simply making an effort to breathe is taken as evidence of brain function. I then finish this line by saying, "If there is no evidence of brain function on either exam and he does not make any effort to breathe, then he will be declared dead."

I complete the protocol description by saying, "We understand that this is your husband, brother and father. So even if he is declared dead, we will not remove the tubes and stop all therapies until you have had time to grieve and be with him. We hope that can be done within a few hours." Requests for more than four hours are discouraged with apologies. Exceptions can be made if reasonable.

Some family members may wish to observe the exam. We permit that but I require that they be sitting because I have had family members faint and fall observing the testing of brainstem reflexes. I also strongly prefer only one observer or two at most.

After each exam or apnea test, the testing physician reports to the family whether there is or is not evidence of brain function and whether the protocol will continue or not. If the family has been educated properly, they know exactly what that means. Family members who witnessed the exam always nod their assent.

It should be obvious that, in most cases that a patient is this sick, the acceptance of brain death is much easier for the family than when there is evidence of brain function. During the meeting, if they ask what happens if there is evidence of brain function, I respond "Then we will have a much harder conversation."

The last related topic is organ donation. Brain death determination is preferred for organ donation because the patient can be maintained physiologically until in the OR and organs are better preserved with better transplant survival rates. If the patient has chosen organ donation or the family has consented to organ donation, then a member of the transplant team or Gift of Life will assume care after declaration of Brain Death. You can see why "Separation" is so important as previously discussed.

Chapter 14. Avoiding Being Judgmental

This brief chapter is devoted to a single common error which I will refer to as "being judgmental." It is a subtle type of error with important negative consequences for our patient relationships. In many ways it is the opposite of feeling compassion for our patients. Certainly it stands in the way of being compassionate. Note that, despite the similarity of the two terms, "being judgmental" is unrelated to the good "judgement" which we have been discussing as essential to our role as physicians.

Being judgmental can be defined as a tendency to form an unfair, usually harsh, opinion about someone's character. In the setting of the doctor-patient relationship, it represents forming an opinion, generally negative and critical, about a person's personality or motivation based on initial observations of their behaviors.

We all have a tendency to do this in everyday life, it is common and natural, but it can interfere with our professional responsibilities to heal.

Being judgmental in medicine is more likely to occur when a patient's disease appears to be related to behaviors with risk of self harm such as addiction to drugs, alcohol or cigarettes. It also occurs when an unhealthy lifestyle, such as sedentary behavior and over-eating, is associated with the patient's condition, especially obesity. At other times, we are judgmental when a patient does not adhere to our recommendations, either because they don't agree with our plan or because they are non-compliant. It also can happen when a patient is not responding to our recommended treatment and both they and we are becoming frustrated.

None of these reasons are fair. We almost never know the background of our patients sufficiently well to understand why they adopted these behaviors. What previous physical or psychological events contributed to their development, including those related to negative experiences during childhood or adolescence? Recent genetic and pharmacological studies have clearly demonstrated that obesity, as well as alcohol and drug abuse, have major genetic components. How can we "blame" someone for that?

Then why do we do it? Studies have identified diverse reasons that include societal conditioning, reinforcement of our own values, the need for control, a way to avoid reckoning with our feelings, and as a defense mechanism for our own insecurities or shortcomings. It is easy to see how these reasons might relate to the conditions described above.

A unique and tragic situation can arise when we encounter a patient who has a borderline personality or is suicidally depressed. Those patients have a tendency to behave in such a manner that they actually stimulate a negative reaction on our part in order to confirm their own negative feelings or beliefs which arise as a consequence of their disorder.

Being judgmental is never useful in medicine and has important negative consequences for the doctor-patient relationship. Patients are aware when physicians are being judgmental. Numerous patients have told me that they refuse to return for follow-up to a physician because they felt that they had been judged unfairly. None of us want that. Our judgmental attitude damages the doctor-patient relationship by promoting distrust, increasing the risk of conflict, and hindering growth of understanding and compassion. It can have direct negative consequences for the patient, contributing to stress, anxiety, and even depression. It tends to perpetuate self-stereotypes and reinforce reactions to discrimination. In patients with pre-existing psychiatric disturbances it may increase their sense of isolation or even the risk of suicide.

Earlier in the book, the point was made that our bedside role includes being the doctor that our patient needs us to be in order to get well.

Being judgmental takes us away from that goal. It prevents us from being the doctor that they need.

Obviously, I am prone to this problem just like everyone else. The only way I have found to address it is to be conscious of the risk, recognize when it is happening and isolate the feeling from my role as a physician. I rely heavily on the saying of Buddha, "Life is so difficult, how can we be anything but kind?" When I reflect on that, it increases my sense of compassion and reorients my mind toward helping my patient recover.

In those patients in whom changes in lifestyle are important, even though I avoid being judgmental, I need to help them change the behaviors with potential for harm. I begin with another saying of Buddha. "Buddha says, 'No matter how difficult the past, we can always begin again today.'" Whether the treatment that is needed is behavioral, pharmacological or procedural, or a combination, my job is to integrate those treatments into a package that helps the patient avoid the previous injurious behaviors over the long term.

If my judgmental behavior is part of a defense mechanism, however, then I must reflect on my own role, ensure that my compassion and professional responsibilities rise above my fears and discomfort, and find the courage to meet the challenge together with the patient.

Buddha is my teacher, I don't know why exactly. You must find your own.

Chapter 15. Making Mistakes

We all make mistakes.

There is no way around this, no one is perfect. One good goal is to try to avoid making the same mistake twice. Another important goal of the medical community is that we learn to share our mistakes with one another in an effort to reduce the number of times that any particular mistake is made by anyone.

It's not easy to share mistakes. Admitting that we have erred, possibly with a negative result for our patients, is uncomfortable and risks loss of stature. There is a great deal involved in this behavior. We have to be confident in ourselves and our ability to learn from our mistakes. We have to avoid judging and criticizing others when they have enough courage to share their mistakes. We have to learn to discuss mistakes in a spirit of growth and dedication to the well being of our patients while overcoming our own egoistical tendencies. It is a culture which must be created and sustained in our universities, medical centers and throughout the medical community.

A surgeon and I were caring for a patient at Stony Brook. The surgeon had operated on her abdomen the day before and she had more pain than expected post-op and a mildly elevated WBC. The surgeon arranged to take her back to the OR. When I asked him why he did not observe her for 24 hours instead, he answered "Based on my experience." He paused and then added, "By 'my experience,' I mean my mistakes."

One key to avoiding unnecessary mistakes is to learn to recognize and acknowledge when you don't know. That may apply to a technical skill that you are assigned. What should you do if you lack that technical skill or do not have confidence in your ability to execute it? Ask for help!

On the ward, I am often amazed as a consultant speaks to our team explaining new ideas in their sub-specialty that are pertinent to the patient. Everyone stands around nodding their head but I am thinking, "We have no idea what he is saying, not really." I assure you that, without any hesitation, I interrupt the consultant and say "I don't mind exposing my ignorance. I don't understand what you're saying. Could you explain this a bit more please?"

A concept of Zen is often translated as "Don't know mind." There are similar quotes from Socrates, Confucius, Abraham Lincoln and StarTrek that state that the beginning of wisdom is to admit that you don't know. It is better to admit that you are ignorant than to remain ignorant. Don't be shy about this, I assure you that I am not.

There are many excellent sources that go into detail about why physicians make mistakes. I recommend that you find one that seems to suit you and read it. One source of error that is particularly disturbing to me is an error related to an unyielding attitude on the part of the physician. The attitude may be due to arrogant overconfidence, or disrespect for another physician's opinion, or pride in the wisdom of one specialty over another specialty, or of judging the patient, or of refusing to acknowledge that a more junior person might have better insight into the present situation, or personal ego, or disregard for a family member's observations. It is daunting to think about how many ways we can get it wrong. But most of these "errors of attitude" share an unwillingness to consider alternatives to our pre-conceived understanding of a situation. We become focused on an idea and no longer permit contrary information to influence our thinking. The exact reason that we ignore the information varies, but the root of the problem is that for reasons which are not based on science or logic we refuse to admit the new information into our reasoning. It is the patient who pays the price, of course. Because the specifics are so diverse, this is a challenging error to avoid, especially during the pressure of daily life caring for patients. Buddha says, "It's not your preferences that get you into trouble, its your attachments to them." I <u>try</u> to avoid this error by admitting my own fallibility and keeping an open mind to alternative ways of thinking. Every idea that is offered deserves my attention and unbiased reflection to see how it can contribute to the care of my patient. It doesn't matter what the source is. Plato said, "If knowledge could come from a tree, should we reject it?"

The best solution to all of these potential errors that I ever heard came during a talk being given by a former head of the Federal Aeronautics Administration. He basically said that reaching the minuscule level of error that is required for a safe air transportation network requires multiple levels of redundancy. To make his point, he said, "If you write an order for something to be done and you just assume it is done without verifying it, then you are a fool."

I often express this inversely. "In order for there to be a screw-up, everyone has to screw up. Because if even one person doesn't screw up, then there is no screw-up." That's why redundancy is so important. Attending, Resident, Student, Nurse, Therapist, Pharmacist, Clerk, Chaplains, and on. Modern medicine of major diseases is simply too complex for any one individual. The best solution is to build a redundant system of independent thinkers and foster a culture of inquiry with open expression of doubt. And to listen. And to think again with an open mind.

But we all make mistakes. We cannot let those mistakes destroy our self-confidence or prevent us from continuing to provide the best care possible to our next patients. Buddha says, "If our compassion does not include ourselves, then it is incomplete."

Chapter 16. Surviving as a student (or junior resident)

One of the most difficult parts of being a medical student or first year resident is the rapid change of services that is a standard part of the experience. No sooner do you get used to how things are done in one discipline than you are off to another. Like a nomad, continuously entering new environments.

I'd like to make a few suggestions for how to reduce the frazzle and help you get the most out of each rotation. Try any or all of these and see if they help.

Become a Member of the Team

Without question, my foremost advice is to become one of the doctors on the team, in every sense of the word. A medical rotation is not only an opportunity to learn more information, it is the best chance you will ever have to learn how the members of that specialty think and to experience what their life is like. While this might help some of you decide if you like the specialty as a career, it is invaluable for everyone as a way of getting into the heads of these doctors. If you do that, you will be MUCH more valuable when you share a patient with them and you will create deeper and richer relationships with your colleagues.

You also earn their respect (and improve your grade). But it really is an invaluable opportunity to "walk in another man's shoes" as the Polish expression goes. You will see how difficult it can be and you will learn what it is that excites these practitioners. Chances are it will also make learning the information easier because you understand what they need to know and why they need to know it in order to care for their patients. You also will learn what it is like for a patient to be treated for one of these problems and that also will help you to help your future patients with similar or related problems, even if you are not the doctor treating them.

You should take some night call with them if you really want to be part of the team, even if it is not required. One or two nights won't hurt but it will add another dimension to your understanding. It also shows them that you are serious about learning what they do and are willing to put in some hard work. You gain all around.

How do you start? Follow the old adage, "When in Rome, do as the Romans do." But how do you know what to do when you first get to Rome? Observe! "You first, please." And then you're off. Have fun!

If at all possible, find a way to be useful. By useful, I mean share the work. Take responsibility for a task that you think you can handle. It might be some simple "scut" like bringing a paper or lab sample somewhere or picking things up or helping to transport a patient. You will be amazed at what you learn. "Places to go, things to do, people to meet." And you become part of the team.

It's also a good idea to be cognizant of when there is time to ask a question of your seniors and attendings. When can you interrupt and when shouldn't you?

Getting to the Key Information for the New Specialty ASAP

Find out from the team members which textbooks and lectures are best at addressing the common disorders and syndromes that occur in this specialty. Read and ask about the syndromes that are seen regularly and focus on the most common syndromes first.

Which features of the history help to differentiate the various common syndromes?

Are there specialized parts of the physical exam which are particularly useful? Get a more senior clinician to help you learn to elicit signs and go see patients who have these findings if possible.

Two funny personal anecdotes. I wanted to be a neurologist by the time I was 12 years old. When I joined the Neurology service as a 3rd year student, I was in hog heaven. One day I heard Neurology paged stat to the floor immediately above me. Without any thought, I ran up and, unfortunately, was the first one there. There was a woman in full opisthotonus, arched such that only her occiput and heels were touching the bed. I had seen pictures so I knew what it was but I had NO IDEA what to do. I felt like an idiot as I asked her if it hurt. (She said no.) Mercifully for both me and the patient, a senior neurology resident arrived within a minute. He just looked at her and asked (in 1974) "Has this patient received compazine?" The nurses affirmed that she had for post-surgical nausea. "Well give her 2 mg of benztropine." And that was that, it was over. Am I sorry that happened? Not in a million years. That was by far the best example that I have ever seen and I learned how to recognize dystonic reactions, and how to manage them, "while still a pup."

In the second story, I was the subject. I was already a Professor of Neurology and Stroke Director at Stony Brook. I was at the head of our team on the ward (I walk quite fast) when I happened to mention that I had a bit of eczema under the eye pieces of my glasses. A very short medical student virtually flew in front of me and we were suddenly stopped, nose to nose. I almost walked right into her. I could, literally, hear the other students behind me gasp. But there I was confronted by this half-crazed young woman trying to see under my glasses. I was tremendously amused. I asked, "Would you like me to take off my glasses?" She nearly melted. I did, she gazed and gazed. Then she sort of went blank, as if to store the images. Then she responded, "Thanks, I'm done" and released me. I loved it! And I loved her for the passion that drove her fearlessly to seek out an opportunity to improve her knowledge and skills as a future dermatologist.

Here's another bit of useful advice. The service's standardized chart notes and admission order sets are another great source to help find out the key elements that you need to learn. The standardized notes distill the information that is most important for diagnosing and managing their patients. The order sets show you the common standing orders as well as the most common labs, electrophysiology and imaging tests that are used. It's a great way to help you identify what you most need to know. Make sure you understand why by asking the more senior residents and by reading on your own. The best reading is usually in review articles or recent textbooks.

Using Systems Biology to Adjust Quickly When You First Enter a Field

The term "systems biology" is recent enough that it is still a fluid concept. For our current purpose, the idea is that you should not be looking for a diagnosis out in the small branches and leaves of the tree until you know that you are on the right limb.

I recommend that your first reading priority for a new field should be to become familiar with the most common clinical syndromes. What type of patient are you likely to see on Day 1? What problems are you likely to be seeing during the rotation?

Next, I suggest that you review the normal anatomy and physiology of the key body organs involved in that field. It's not a bad idea to do that the night before you start.

Then I would review the mechanisms of disease that affect the central organs of the discipline. Mechanisms of disease is synonymous with Pathophysiology. While I am not a big fan of memorizing lists, the list of pathophysiologic mechanisms is one list that I absolutely do recommend that you memorize. This list includes all mechanisms that can produce disease states.

1. Vascular
2. Trauma
3. Infectious
4. Inflammatory
5. Neoplastic
6. Psychiatric
7. Metabolic
8. Toxic
9. Genetic

10. Degenerative
11. Ambient energy disturbances (including ionizing radiation)

This last category includes things like photon radiation (including sun and X-rays); blast, sound and ultrasound; heat and cold; and prolonged exposure to water and extreme dryness.

One of the values of knowing this list is that the mechanisms and clinical characteristics of each category tend to be relatively constant from one organ system to the next. Organized around these mechanisms, what you learn in one medical field tends to carry over considerably into other fields. There are unique features among the organ systems, of course, but the time course of presentation, presence of pain, and events that trigger the presentation of each disease mechanism tend to be similar from one system to the next.

Finally, knowing the common syndromes, the normal anatomy and physiology, and relevant mechanisms of disease, you are ready to associate each of the common syndromes with the most common etiologies so that you can formulate a reasonable differential diagnosis early in your rotation. The list of disease mechanisms, which will already be familiar to you from prior rotations, serves as a valuable mnemonic aid as you review the possible specific etiologies for your patient´s syndrome.

You have my sincere condolences! This rotation from one new system to the next is tiring. Over and over, the cycle involves reading well into the night your first week on a new service and then continuous literature searching for the rest of the rotation. It is important that you learn to use the literature efficiently. Modern search tools are awesome. If it is any comfort to you, on an average day, I do about 15 literature searches. I use them to fill holes in my basic and medical knowledge as well as to assure that my patient management knowledge is up to date. A whole chapter has been devoted to this important tool that you will use throughout your career. You will have to learn to integrate AI into your practice on your own. I'll be no help to you there.

Competency VI - Systems

I use this term mildly tongue in cheek but it is actually quite important. The idea is that you need to learn how to participate in a healthcare system, eventually as one of its leaders. My advice to you is based on many years of leading medical teams of varied sizes, from a few people to several thousand people. This is what I have learned about running a medical center.

Rule #1. Look up and say Hello. Don't be looking down all time. Eyes front! And then make eye contact, and then give a nod or simple acknowledgment. Do it all day long, everywhere you go.

Rule #2. Learn as many first names as possible. Or last names, as is appropriate. The first time you work with someone, anyone, introduce yourself and ask their name. Say "Hi" and repeat their name so it reaches at least to your thalamus. Look at them so you associate the face with the name. Then work together. Then say "Thanks, {name}. Nice working with you."

Rule #3. Help whenever possible, I mean, whenever. Hold the door open for someone carrying something or pushing a wheelchair, help the transport staff turn stretchers, they know how to do it alone but it is much easier if someone will prevent the tail end from moving laterally. Reduces damage to hospital doors as well. You can pick things up but you also need to be mindful of Universal Precautions, you don't want to contaminate yourself or others. I keep two gloves in an inside pocket of my white coat for this purpose. If a nurse is trying to do three things at once, ask if you can help, maybe just by watching the patient or going and asking another nurse to bring something that is needed. There are so many little things that make everyone's life easier and more pleasant. And, in the heat of action, it just feels good to know that someone sees you as a person and is willing to help.

Getting Things Done in a Timely Manner

When you need something done, especially in a specific time frame, there are several things to do. Remember the FAA consultant's comment. First, make sure the order has been entered, and in the proper manner. I can't tell you how many times I call the tech for an MRI that I am waiting for and hear her respond, "Oh, that was cancelled because they didn't fill out the screening form." The resident swears that they did, and I believe them. But there is no request in the system. So you have to confirm that there is an order!

Next, go to the person or lab or team that will be performing the task. Then ask politely if it can be done in the time frame that you need and, immediately and without pausing, explain why it is important for the patient that it be done within that time frame. Patient care is the key to medicine. It is why we do what we do. It is our purpose. Everyone in medicine responds best to the needs of patient care.

Everyone in the medical center thought that I was able to get things done amazingly quickly because I was a Chairman. That is emphatically wrong. I go to the people who have to perform the procedure, whether doctor, nurse, tech, clerk transport, janitor, chaplain or any other position. I know almost everyone by name. I treat everyone with respect and learn everything I can from them. I always limit the work that I request to the minimum necessary to achieve the immediate goal and do everything I can to streamline things for them. I always explain how it helps the patient and why the time frame is important. I thank them beforehand. I attend the procedure, if I can, to emphasize how important it is. I thank them again afterwards and I share the results of the procedure and how it will affect the patient's care and then I give them follow-up. That's not as hard as it sounds. Like so many other things, it takes more awareness than effort. This paragraph has a lot of "I"s but that was on purpose. It is because I do these things that I can get things done so efficiently. That is what I have learned about running a medical center and about how to enhance its excellence. You lead by example.

Recognizing Talent

When you embed yourself in your medical center, you will encounter individual staff members who "go above and beyond." Not only are they skilled at what they do, they do it "with a will" and in a pleasant and efficient manner. They might occupy any position at all. When you run into such a person, you should find a way to acknowledge them. At first, simply introduce yourself, ask who they are and let them know you are impressed with how they function.

As you gain experience, you will get comfortable doing more.

My best friend and hospital HR guru Elliott Kellman and I have found that there are three things that leaders need to do to foster institutional excellence.

1. Make sure that each person is focused on their own career development and advancement.
2. If a person can tell you what makes their work more difficult and it can be fixed, do everything you can to get it fixed.
3. Make sure that everyone knows the Vision and Mission of the medical center and their unit.

I want to focus here on the first of these three. When you encounter a talented person, if you can, if it is appropriate for your and their situation, ask if they are studying to move into a more advanced field. If they are not already, gently encourage them to do so. Let them know that you see them as really talented and with a lot of potential. If they already are studying and it is in healthcare, ask if they intend to stay at your medical center. If they do, ask if you can put in a good word for them. You may think that your recommendation won't help but you would be very, very wrong. Hiring staff is not easy and a positive observation by a "disinterested party" can make the difference between getting or not getting the position for that person. Anyway, you are trying to help your medical center hire the best people, right? Ask who is their supervisor, and let them know you intend to put in a good word. Make a friend while you're at it. Make someone feel good about themself. There is no downside.

Can I Take Responsibility for this Patient in an Emergency?

One last topic before we leave this chapter. Can you lend assistance in a medical emergency? I mean, should you step in and administer emergency aid? Can you be held responsible for a bad outcome? Can you be sued? Is it all right to lend a hand or even lead a resuscitation effort or try to stabilize a patient with minor or major injury?

The answer is that you should do everything that you can to help, especially if you are the most experienced person there or if you can help a more experienced person, typically another doctor, a policeman, fireman or EMS tech. The Good Samaritan laws of every state protects you, even as a medical student, and ensures that you are not liable.

Here are some words from an online source for you to consider that seem reasonable as guidelines. "Good Samaritan laws protect medical personnel, including students, from liability if they provide assistance in an emergency. Medical students aren't bound by the same ethical obligations as qualified doctors, but they should still help if they feel able to do so. They should also consider the limits of their experience and knowledge."

An example: Many of our adult Neurology residents are reluctant to treat a child with a neurologic emergency because their training and license are restricted to patients 18 and over. That makes no sense to me. If you are the most capable person present at the site of an emergency, then any effort is better than none at all or the efforts of a person with less knowledge and experience than you. Again, the Good Samaritan laws provide firm legal protection.

So, please, if you find yourself at the site of an emergency, help in the most effective manner that you can. Simply do your best to stabilize the patient, observe carefully and report what you saw and what was done to the EMS personnel so they can pass that information along to the emergency room.

Chapter 17. Learn to Teach

One of the precepts of the Hippocratic Oath is that all physicians are obligated to pass on their knowledge and experience to other doctors. That is, we all must teach one another. In addition, an enormous part of patient care requires patient education so they understand the reason and manner of compliance.

As a result, most residencies include learning to teach as part of their curriculum. At Einstein, there were explicit exercises that the residents needed to do and explicit goals organized by year of training as well as by the venue of teaching, from the bedside to Grand Rounds. Opportunities for teaching non-medical people in the community is strongly encouraged and opportunities that come to the faculty are shared with the residents.

It would be a mistake to think that only those who remain in academic medical centers or university settings need to learn to teach. In some ways, the opposite is true. At academic centers there are many people to share teaching responsibilities and it is possible to "carve out" sub-speciality areas for teaching as well as for practice. But in private healthcare facilities, and especially in smaller ones in more remote settings, the opportunity for specialization does not exist. A neurologist, for example, would need to be able to cover everything, including stroke, neuromuscular disorders, cognitive disorders, sleep, pregnancy, and anything else relevant to the facility staff.

Thus we all need to learn to teach effectively.

A common way of introducing medical students to teaching is the "5 minute talk." Typically, a topic comes up on rounds that is not well understood by members of the team. The Attending or Senior Resident sees the teaching opportunity and assigns it to a medical student, either because it was their patient or because it was "their turn." The point of this is to review the basic and clinical materials that are relevant, using primary literature or systematic reviews more than textbook material, and then develop a background and application to share with everyone. The presentation should last no more than 5 minutes. The topic and organization should be clear from the start. The background should be understandable by all and strictly relevant. The immediate application depends on why the issue arose in the first place and should certainly include a relationship to the patient being discussed. In 5 minutes!

It is also common to assign patient education tasks to medical students, either for their own patients or for a patient who lacks a student. The "pitch" has to be appropriate for the patient's educational level. You will need to know from their history or ask the patient directly. A rule of thumb is to start at the 5th grade educational level and then increase the level of sophistication based on the educational level achieved by the patient. It is nearly always useful to provide the patient with written or graphic material and I like to draw in front of the patient as well, often on the printed materials. They are unlikely to remember everything you tell them so the printed materials provide a way for them to review and share with their family members. Finally, make sure that you have covered the questions that they have, that you have been clear enough for them to understand and to let them know that you will come back tomorrow to see if they have any further questions. If they are being discharged, encourage them to ask their primary provider if they have further questions. It is worthwhile to have them bring the printed materials to their PCP at the first follow-up visit after a hospitalization so that the primary provider knows what was considered important for the patient to know.

Finally, get out into the community. Some of the very best experiences I have ever had as a doctor were out in the community. My first week of internship I volunteered to work that Sunday morning at a VFW blood drive. When I walked in, a large man said "Hi, want some pancakes, Doc?" I nearly fell over. The sound of this big WWII veteran calling me "Doc" was one of the greatest feelings I have ever known. To this day, this computer, my skis and my cameras are all labeled "Doc."

Other great opportunities included speaking to the Hmong about stroke. The Hmong are a community of mountain dwellers from Vietnam who have no written language. I learned that their translators can mentally record at least 15 minutes of speech and translate from English to Hmong seemingly effortlessly. And then there was the time that I lectured on stroke to a Black Baptist Church in Philadelphia using the theme "Am I my brother's keeper?" You may think that the pastor drives the congregation in the increasing intensity that you have seen on TV, but that experience taught me the power of the congregation to drive the speaker. OMG, what a feeling!

There is a richness to the world that is available to you through the ethnic groups in your community based on your capacity as healer and teacher. I strongly encourage you to avail yourself of that privilege. The more you do, the more you grow, the better you will get and the better you will be able to serve your patients, your community and your medical center.

Chapter 18. Writing Notes

After face to face communication, note writing is the most important way that we have of communicating our thoughts about our patients. It is the primary way that we have to record and memorialize our ideas and actions. This chapter is limited to a few comments based on observations of how others write notes, how my own notes are received by others and problems that have occurred because of notes. It also builds on over thirty years of my medicolegal chart reviews, reports and testimonies. As for most of the topics in this book, it is not a "how to" recipe book but rather focused suggestions The chapter focuses exclusively on clinical patient notes and does not address other types of notes that pertain to procedures or diagnostic reports (think H&P's and progress notes).

For Whom Do We Write Our Notes?

It's a toss-up in my mind as to whether the primary "recipient" of the note is other medical providers or myself. It is important to keep both in mind. The referring doctor has asked a question or presented a problem. It is our responsibility to provide an opinion regarding that question or problem and to explain in adequate detail what is the basis of our opinion. In that sense, the note is clearly for the referring doctor. But it is usually the case that I will be seeing the patient a second time and, when I do, I will want that second visit to be focused, efficient and sensitive to any changes in history or exam. In that sense, the note is for myself. Throughout the time that I am writing the note, I am conscious that I am communicating with the referring doctor now as well as with myself in the future.

Of course there are many others who may be reading the note for many reasons. But the chances are that if I have written a note that properly serves the referring doctor and myself, anyone else will be able to appreciate what I am saying. Hopefully, I have been thorough enough and clear enough that they will be able to find what they need.

I have a simple piece of advice for doctors seeking to build their practice. Write useful notes! If you do, you will be asked back again. Provide the best answer you can to the referring question or to the patient's primary complaint if you are a primary care physician. Explain and support your opinion. Consider alternative options for diagnosis and management and explain the relative advantages and disadvantages of each possibility. Be clear, avoid a dogmatic approach, specify areas of uncertainty and how best to "fill in the blanks" and provide education by discussing ideas that may be accepted in your field but unfamiliar to someone outside your sub-specialty. In other words, leave a useful note. I want to emphasize this last point. Thoughtful, succinct discussions in your notes are an invaluable means of educating other physicians. Put another way, a major goal of your note should be to have the reader look forward to the next time they can work with you. By writing a useful note, and by direct conversation, is how you build a big practice. And a big practice is useful whether you are in private practice or whether you are in academics, where you want people to involve you so that your residents and students have a lot of patients to learn from.

The SOAP Note

For your notes to be useful, not only must your thinking be clear but the organization of your note has to make it clear, easy to read and easy to navigate so that the information and logic are easily available. Given that we are in the era of EMR, I will leave out any comments about the legibility of your handwriting, like the good old days when we used to have to find someone "who could read Henry's writing."

There are many ways of organizing notes but when students ask me for advice on how to organize their note, I always recommend beginning with "SOAP." It is just a great way of reaching the clarity discussed above. There are many other approaches that work, most of which embed SOAP implicitly or explicitly, so why not start with that basic?

SOAP refers, of course, to **S**ubjective, **O**bjective, **A**ssessment and

Plan. Note that this is not quite the same as "History and Physical" although there is overlap. Why not? First of all, because a History is obtained from many sources, not just the patient, and includes information from other people as well as prior medical records. Therefore the term "Subjective" is not the appropriate term, literally speaking. It serves the purpose, however, as long as you keep the larger context in mind.

Conversely, "Objective" refers to a much larger data set than "Exam" because, although it includes the exam and vital signs, it also includes laboratory data, electrophysiology (EKG, EEG, etc.) and imaging. Again, there is no harm here as long as this is kept in mind.

Let's just make this clear. The "S" subsumes all of the information that you obtain from others. This includes the patient's history as well as input from other witnesses and from available factual materials which likely include notes from physicians and other practitioners who have seen the patient previously. The "O" refers to the information that you, yourself, can observe and evaluate, either by examining the patient or reviewing available lab results or images as well as the reports. Whether you put prior labs, electrophysiology and imaging in the subjective section or objective section depends primarily on where the placement best contributes to the logical argument that you are trying to develop as you try to explain how the patient has reached the present state.

Happily, the terms "Assessment" and "Plan" are perfectly adequate, although a few brief comments are in order. The "Assessment" should include your differential diagnosis along with a highlight of the data pertinent to the differential. If you've already covered details of labs, etc., you can just refer to them briefly in this section, indicating how they contribute to your differential. There is nearly always need for a brief discussion around the differential diagnosis indicating the relative probability of each item and their inter-relationships. This is the primary opportunity in your note for education.

In Neurology, the etiologic Differential Diagnosis should be preceded by a discussion of the localization within the nervous system that best explains the patients complaints and findings, including alternative localizations when appropriate. That way, the localization can guide the etiologic differential diagnosis in a logical manner.

The Plan includes your recommendations either to the patient or to the referring doctor for further diagnostic testing as needed to complete unanswered questions pertinent to localization, etiology, prognosis and subsequent management. The Plan also includes recommendations for immediate treatments to help ameliorate bothersome symptoms and to slow the disease process if there is already adequate certainty of the diagnosis, that is, if your judgement has crossed the Treatment Threshold. The plan should include long-term management including recommendations for other consults that may be useful and who should assume responsibility for each aspect of the patient's care. Finally, this section usually also includes a brief notation on what was said to the patient and family so that other practitioners seeing the patient will know what has already been discussed. There is usually opportunity for education here as well.

One thing that I find missing from the SOAP note structure is an introduction to the patient which should really be the very first part of the note but is based on your observations and not on subjective data. I tell students who are presenting a patient to me that I want to be able to "see" the patient that they are talking about even though I haven't actually met the patient yet. I believe that should be the opening of each note on a new patient. For example, "The patient is a 67 year old white woman, looking her stated age. She was neatly dressed and attentive but appeared anxious and was tearful at several points in the history." That is my only suggestion for modifying the basic SOAP note. Some include this type of information early in "O."

I recognize all of this is easy to say, and I'm trying to keep it concise here. But there is no question that these short paragraphs "are a mouthful." It takes a lot of work, coordination and practice to complete all of these tasks properly.

The Problem Oriented Medical Record (POMR)

The POMR is another useful system for organizing notes in the medical record. As you will see, the SOAP note fits well into the POMR. The POMR is a higher level of organization than a single note and pertains to the patient's entire chart (in the EMR).

The basic components of the POMR are:

- Data Base - History, Physical Exam and Laboratory Data (in the SOAP note)
- Complete Problem List
- Initial Plans (also part of the SOAP note)
- Daily Progress Note (Can follow a simplified SOAP format without headings)
- Final Progress Note (SOAP format) or Discharge Summary which is usually specific for the medical center and service

How you interact with the Problem List is a function of the EMR but it is often confusing and simply ends up a part of the billing apparatus. Depending on how your EMR is structured, it may or may not be inserted into your note. If it isn't, it is the responsibility of the primary team to maintain an up-to-date problem list. It is rarely clear how consultants should participate in the Problem List. Last time I looked, an accurate problem list remains an unfulfilled wish in most EMR's although some integrated healthcare systems such as Kaiser Permanente, Mayo Clinic and Geisinger Clinic may come pretty close.

Follow-up notes are generally a shorter version of the initial note with similar structure, except in the ICU where new and follow-up notes are pretty similar in length. I use headings for the SOAP sections in my initial note but rarely in a follow-up note. In follow-up notes, paragraphs with double hard returns are used more commonly to separate the sections.

Some Specific Issues

Many services have developed specific formats for progress notes that facilitate recording and communicating the most relevant information for their practices. These are useful to all and, as previously discussed, excellent tools for learning. So ask about them when you rotate onto a new service but also check if it is appropriate for you to use them since you don't want to introduce duplication in the EMR.

ICU teams nearly always have pre-specified formats for their notes. However, even within one medical center, the surgical, medical and specialized ICU's may all have unique note formats. Usually, ICU notes follow a fairly explicit organ system approach. This usually includes some version of the SOAP format for each system, usually along with relevant vital signs, the presence of indwelling tubes, connected devices and current medications, as well as anticipated or recently completed procedures. This format can be helpful outside the ICU for any complex hospitalized patient.

You will often refer to other services in your notes. This requires a bit of sensitivity. Most obviously, you need to be accurate in referring to their findings, opinions and recommendations. Unless there is a reason to refer to one specific physician, it is usual to refer to the service, not a doctor by name. That acknowledges both the involvement of a whole team as well as providing leeway for physician rotations. If a specific doctor is playing a central role, however, then it is appropriate to include the name of that doctor.

There will be many times when the Plan is uncertain. A particular invasive test may be under consideration but not yet decided upon, possibly because the need for the test will be determined by the patient's response to ongoing treatment. A simple acknowledgment of the uncertainty is usually adequate, "Will consider biopsy if patient does not respond to current management" will do fine. When you are discussing a possible procedure performed by another service, or are not even sure which procedure would be most efficacious, and that service has not yet included a specific recommendation in their notes or has not yet even been consulted, a statement such as "Will discuss with Cardiology" is appropriate. If the service isn't even certain, a note such as "Need for coronary procedures under discussion."

It is usual to include some acknowledgment of the referring doctor or medical center, along with the specific reason for referral. "Ms. Jones was referred by Dr. Smith of Valley Forge for evaluation of progressive weight loss with intermittent fever." This can be logically placed early in the Subjective portion of the SOAP note.

This also requires a bit of sensitivity since referral implies the need for assistance, the doctor or medical center has not solved the problem on their own. It is important to avoid the implication of criticism in your note if you want to receive more referrals from them in the future. There is no reason for any of that anyway, think of it as not being judgmental. Use of the passive voice can be helpful when there are genuine concerns about events prior to arrival. For example, "The patient continued to deteriorate despite treatment and . . ." We all find ourselves over our heads and need to reach out to others for help at some point. Everyone wants their patient to improve. "There is no They, there is only We."

Notes for Diagnostic and Therapeutic Procedures

I don't do procedures, and so I don't write procedural notes. But I do read them and so am writing this for all of you future proceduralists with the ulterior motive of making the lives of us clinicians easier.

Procedural notes usually have separate technical and interpretative sections. I read both sections for procedures done on my patients. I read the technical section to learn but also to identify unexpected findings during the procedure. For me, unexpected findings in one of my patients is an important learning opportunity. Why didn't I anticipate that finding? Was there some clinical data which might have helped me recognize that before the procedure? That is important for my future patients. Also, unexpected findings often mean that the originally planned procedure had to be modified. This may place the patient at risk for future complications including failure of the procedure or infection. So I always read the technical section.

A well-written interpretative section of a diagnostic procedure addresses the clinical question. On the one hand, the relevant specific findings derived from the test, both positive and negative, need to be stated. Then these findings should be associated with potential organ pathophysiology and etiology based on the diagnostician's experience and knowledge of the literature. Just as for clinical notes, a differential diagnosis with some estimate of probability is desirable. A sense of probability is particularly useful in notes from Radiologists and microscopic Pathologists.

That said, my experience has been that additional insight into a diagnostic test, especially electrophysiology and imaging, can be gained if I speak with the diagnostician after the test. They simply never put all of their uncertainties and concerns in their note. Also, they rarely have all of the clinical information regarding the patient. Therefore, especially when dealing with complex patients, a discussion between the diagnostician and the treating clinician should be standard. I simply cannot state this strongly enough. It should be part of your routine. You are doing the study to answer a question. Don't you want the best answer possible? And the discussion should be documented in your next progress note. Radiologists nearly explode with joy when they hear me say this.

Medicolegal Concerns About Your Notes

This is simple! Basically, a good medical note is a good medicolegal note. That's all there is to it. Be clear about your actions, explicit about your thoughts and decision making, document your uncertainties, concerns and discussions with other physicians. Avoid judgmental comments and "chart wars." Nothing new there, that's your best defense in the event of any legal action.

The next chapter takes up additional medicolegal issues.

Chapter 19. Medicolegal Issues

This is a topic which causes great Angst but need not if you follow a few simple principles.

We have already addressed medicolegal issues of note writing and Good Samaritan laws. To summarize them succinctly, a well-written clinical note covers all of the important medicolegal issues and the Good Samaritan laws provide you with the legal coverage that you need to render emergency care to the best of your abilities.

This chapter will address a few medicolegal circumstances which you might encounter as a student or resident.

Morbidity and Mortality Conferences

The closest thing to legal scrutiny that we routinely encounter in medicine is the M&M, the Morbidity and Mortality conference. This is a valuable form of QI in which patient care is reviewed with the goal of identifying opportunities for improvement and exploring alternative management strategies. Cases may be chosen for M&M because of an unanticipated untoward outcome, or because the case provides a good example for learning or because of a pre-determined selection schema. In addition to all of the benefits that a thorough review can provide for future medical care, it also represents an excellent vehicle for learning what a medical record really looks like when viewed at high mag. You will be surprised at what you see.

Although the purposes (and the consequences) of chart review for an M&M and medicolegal purposes are different, the methodology is quite similar. In both cases, it is desirable for the reviewer to be critical, fair and precise in the assessment of the chart. By "critical" I do not mean with the intent to criticize but rather to review with the highest possible standards. Nothing should be assumed during the review. As the saying goes, "If it isn't documented, it didn't happen." For both the M&M and medicolegal reviews, the initial review is intended to understand the sequence of events that transpired and to understand the reasoning and decisions that were made by the physicians. Were they seeking the correct information, were they using that information wisely, did they have the necessary knowledge and experience to care for the patient and ability to seek help if they did not? Were any actions taken that most practitioners would have done differently? If there were actions that were not within the usual standards, were those actions justified by notations of why the standard approach was not applicable for this patient? Were there opportunities to improve? Was there harm to the patient as a result of the treating teams' actions? Were there unresolved differences of opinions among the treating physicians evident in the medical record? Were there recommendations or plans that were neither followed nor "excused?" These and similar questions form the basis of both the M&M and the medicolegal review.

Also, both types of reviews usually lead to summary reports and the two types of reports have similar structure. In both cases, the data learned from chart review is presented succinctly, usually in chronological sequence. Any differences of findings or interpretations observed upon inspection of available electrophysiology or imaging by the reviewer from those in the medical record are noted, a short, relevant review of pertinent literature is provided, and then a summary assessment, including variations from standards and possible alternative management strategies, is provided. In both types of reports, the first goal is accuracy and the second is clarity. A good report is free of emotional comments. Good lawyers say that they don't like it when an expert uses an exclamation point. A well-written report should stand up to scrutiny by others and, ideally, should not contain even one single statement that needs to be retracted. Don't overreach. Stay centered on the facts and be fair in all assessments.

Of course, the two reports differ significantly in their usage. The M&M is to improve future patient care by those involved in the patient management, by those who conduct the review and by those who participate in the conference discussion. The medicolegal report is used by the requesting lawyer to decide whether to institute or continue legal proceedings and to develop a strategy to prove or refute a claim of injury due to negligence in front of a jury.

A comprehensive study of medical malpractice highlighted three major findings. First, most lawsuits related to alleged malpractice did not involve malpractice. Second, most cases of malpractice never result in lawsuits. Third, for there to be a big jury settlement there must be three factors present. There was negligence, there was injury and the defense was arrogant.

Being Part of Your Medical Center's Legal Team

It will not take you long to learn when there is a potential law suit for negligence. When there is an unexpected poor patient outcome, or an unanticipated complication of a procedure, especially when there has been friction between one or more family members and the medical team, or if a family member overtly threatens legal action, then there is the potential for legal action.

What should be your response? Three things. First, you should make sure that your medical center's risk management office is notified immediately, either by you or by a more senior member of your team. Secondly, you should not discuss this matter with anyone outside of the immediate treating team, your supervisors or the responsible management of your medical center. Third, if there is to be a review of the patient's management by the hospital, do it within an M&M or QI setting, or in conjunction with your lawyers, so that people may speak freely without fear of disclosure in court. This is being challenged in state courts as I write this but M&M and QI conferences remain exempt from disclosure as far as I am aware.

You should not discuss this with anyone outside of your medical center. You should not respond to requests from lawyers, orally or written, unless they come from your medical center's own legal office. You should not attempt to dissuade the family from seeking legal advice. However, even if you are sympathetic to their situation, you should not say or write anything that implies that there has been improper care. Such statements will be inaccurately repeated and used against your colleagues.

You should continue to care for the patient to the best of your ability and treat the family the same way you would have if there was no threat of legal action. Simply go about your usual business of being the patient's doctor. That's actually easier than you would expect, just think "medically." If there is a significant rift with the family, sufficient to interfere with good joint decision making, then it is appropriate to acknowledge to the family that "you appear to have lost confidence in our team" and ask if they would like to consider having the patient transferred to another medical center, assuming the patient is sufficiently stable to tolerate transfer.

If transfer is requested in the setting of patient or family dissatisfaction, then who should make the arrangements for transfer varies among medical centers? A key issue is who seeks an accepting physician, the patient or the medical team, as well as who pays the cost of transfer. Clearly, if the patient's problems require services that are not available in your medical center then your team becomes responsible to find an accepting medical center and arranges transport. The medical center pays for transport. However, if your medical center has the capability to care for the patient's problems but the family is dissatisfied, then many medical centers require that the family is responsible to find an accepting team at another medical center and is responsible for costs of transfer (which may be considerable). Obviously this criteria is not black and white, so there will need to be discussions that should involve your Attending and, in most cases, senior management of the medical center. Also, sometimes there are alternative treating teams within your medical center and transfer to another service may satisfy the family, avoiding the risks of transferring a potentially unstable patient.

Are these situations messy? You bet they are! No one feels good about them. Unfortunately, they happen from time to time and have to be addressed. We need to act in a professional manner and minimize the role of any personal feelings. Buddha says, "Learn to respond and not to react." Following that maxim and acting professionally usually yields the best strategies for these difficult situations. It may help you to have and show more compassion if you remember that you are the professional and that the family is tremendously stressed and aggrieved by the illness of their loved one. Don't take it personally.

Depositions

It is certainly possible that you will be asked to participate in a deposition as a resident. It would be unusual to have a student participate. There are several points worth making regarding depositions.

It is likely that you would receive a letter saying that you have been subpoenaed to participate in a deposition. You may also receive a demand for you to provide all of your records and answer a long list of questions, known as "Interrogatories." All of that sounds scary, especially the "subpoena" and long list of "Interrogatories." Your response should be to calmly contact the legal office of your medical center and show them what you have received. From that point on you will be guided by your legal team. They will explain all that you need to know about attending the deposition and THEY will complete the Interrogatories. You do not. They are likely to discuss the questions with you, however. After discussion between your lawyers and the opposing lawyers, they will decide whether you really do or do not need to participate in the deposition.

Let's make a list of things that need to be clear about depositions. You might want to use this section, indeed this whole chapter, as a reference and return to it if you ever are deposed rather than read it now. There is no harm at all in moving on to the next chapter from this point. But in case you are deposed, here is a list of facts and suggestions that you are likely to find very useful.

1. Your deposition has been initiated by the opposing lawyer.
2. Depositions can take place in person or remotely if in person is inconvenient for either side. It is unusual for a factual witness to have to travel, especially when the factual witness is a doctor with active responsibilities. The legal teams travel.
3. Your role is to serve as a factual or "evidentiary" witness. Expert witnesses are hired by the legal teams and that's not going to happen during your training. So your testimony will be limited to explaining what happened to the patient. Topics such as "causation" and "standards of care" are relevant to the experts, not to you. Your lawyer at the deposition will object and instruct you not to answer any question about anything other than factual information.
4. The deposing lawyer has complete control over what parts of your testimony are used after the deposition, including at trial if there is one. It is necessary for you to understand this. In other words, you CANNOT "score points" in a deposition but you can provide information that may be useful to the opposing lawyer if you are not careful. If the lawyer doesn't like what you said then they simply will not introduce your statements as evidence, even if your answer was "true." Given that, your strategy in a deposition is entirely defensive. Your lawyer will let you know what that means for your particular case.
5. It is ESSENTIAL that you prepare thoroughly with your legal team through a series of meetings before the deposition. Ideally, these meetings are two way streets where you and your legal team share perspectives and knowledge. Don't be passive!
    a. At the first meeting, your lawyer will simply ask you questions to determine your understanding and recollection of the events related to the case. You will be provided with relevant parts of the medical record and asked what they mean to you as well as what else you might recall. You should respond thoroughly and honestly.
    b. At a second meeting, your lawyer will bring you up to date on the "big picture" emerging in the case and ask you how you would respond to certain questions. You may be surprised to

learn that there are many honest ways to answer a question. Most importantly, you need to recognize when there are assumptions that have not been justified, and avoid expressing certainty when it isn't justified, or implying complete uncertainty when what you really mean is that one interpretation is much more likely than others but unproven. Your lawyer will suggest alternative ways of answering some of the questions. If they make sense, then that is fine. If you don't understand or agree with the alternative, this is the time to say so. Your lawyer may not love your response but they will NEVER ask you to lie or even say something with which you are uncomfortable. They may suggest alternative ways of expressing your understanding. You must be comfortable with their suggestions or let them know if you are not. It is not useful to make your position better or worse than the facts justify, you only appear dishonest and partisan to a jury.

c. I believe that there should be a third meeting, the night before or morning of your testimony. That provides you with one last opportunity to ask your questions and confirm information. I mentioned earlier that I have experience as an expert witness, I actually like the medicolegal process and have found juries capable of excellent judgements when they are properly educated by the experts. My experience has taught me that preparation with your lawyer is the most important determinant in how well things go at depositions or in trials. There should be no surprises at the deposition if there has been thorough preparation. If there has been good preparation, then after your deposition the deposing lawyer may have additional accurate information about the facts of the case, but nothing else.

6. The deposing lawyer will give you some instructions before the deposition starts. These are benign. If you need a break, say so, although you will have to answer any question that is "pending." If you do not understand a question, ask them to re-state it. If you feel that you need to review the medical record, say so. That sort of thing.

7. A couple of important good practices that you should follow may or may not be part of the instructions.
   a. When asked if you remember something, tell them what you actually remember. If you don´t remember at all, that´s OK, just say "I don't remember." DO NOT GUESS! They may specifically tell you that they don't want you to guess.
   b. Sometimes you may not remember for this patient but the question has to do with a routine that you follow without variation on nearly ever occasion, such as the sequence of your exam. You might not remember examining this patient, but your physical exam for a new patient never varies. So you don´t recall your exam of this patient but you could testify about your "usual practice." As for what you found on exam, you refer to the medical record.
   c. NEVER speculate. "Well, he probably meant to . . ." Nada de eso! Don´t do it.
8. Listen to every question carefully. First of all, is it logical? Would Aristotle approve? Secondly, does it conform with the facts of medicine? Third, does it avoid assumptions that have not been established to this point in the deposition? If the answer to any of these questions is "No" then don´t answer the question. All you need to say is that you cannot answer the question "as asked," and ask them to please re-state the question. If after re-statement the question is still unacceptable, either your lawyer will intervene to help gain clarity or the deposing lawyer may ask you why you can´t answer. You can answer that question and then they can rephrase their question in a manner that avoids your concern.
9. At times during the deposition, your lawyer may object. It actually `happens a lot. Broadly, there are two types of objections. There are purely legal objections about form and other items, and then there are more serious objections which indicate that your lawyer does not want you to answer the pending question. You will not know immediately which is which so, if you hear your lawyer "Object," then stop dead in your tracks, mid word. Either your lawyer will end their objection with "You can answer" or

there will be a discussion between the lawyers. Listen carefully to any discussion that follows, you may gain some insight into your lawyer's concern with the question, including a potential trap or distortion of your opinion. Sit quietly waiting for the dust to settle and to hear <u>your lawyer</u> say "You may answer if you can." Keep your response simple and honest, but be aware of the concerns raised during the discussion. If instructed not to answer by your lawyer, then you do not.

10. The best approach to answering questions is to follow the advice that is given for answering a child's question. "Keep it simple and keep it honest." It's not at all that the person asking is simple. They are not. The point is that you should be absolutely honest in responding but you should not provide more information than is necessary to answer the question.
11. Do not let a deposing lawyer coerce you into admitting something that you do not believe to be correct. They may ask the question multiple times and in several similar ways, but if you don′t like the question or don′t agree with what they are asking, then they cannot force you to say so and your lawyer doesn′t want you to agree out of exhaustion.
12. Do not take on any attitude other than that of a calm, caring physician. Defiance, defensiveness, protectiveness and similar attitudes only dilute your effectiveness by making you appear biased.
13. At times, you may be asked "hypothetical" questions, even though you are a factual witness and not an expert. Hypothetical questions are virtually always incomplete. Your lawyer may object and prohibit you from answering. If they allow it, you can answer the hypothetical, if you are comfortable with it, BUT I would ALWAYS preface my answer with "Given that incomplete hypothetical situation . . ." and I would end my response with " . . . but that doesn't necessarily apply to this patient." Don't even bother with "because . . .", it just doesn't apply.
14. If asked a question with "All things being equal, " I would respond that you have never seen two patients who were the same, so I can't answer that." If asked about "authoritative

sources" such as textbooks or journals, I would respond that no one source is always the best for all situations." These types of questions are the introduction to tricks that will be used to paint you into a corner that you don't want to be in. Better to avoid being corralled in the first place.

15. You will have virtually no communication with your lawyer during the deposition until the "Indirect" portion at the end, after the deposing lawyer has finished. Your lawyer may ask you specific questions based on your responses to questions that have already been addressed in the deposition. They cannot introduce new topics. LISTEN CAREFULLY! There is a reason they are asking that particular question. Likely they feel that you have been unclear or left the wrong implication with your earlier response and want to clarify or delimit what you meant so that your response cannot be mis-interpreted and used at a later time to make a point that you did not intend. Think back to your prep meetings and previous discussions in an effort to understand the reason for their question. Take your time and think, no rush.
16. I always create one very simple form of non-verbal communication with my lawyer before the deposition. I specify a non-verbal sign, such as removing my glasses. If they see that sign then it means that I am not happy with my response to the question that I just finished answering and that I want them to return to THAT immediately preceding question during Indirect. There is no other information that I have ever exchanged during a deposition but I find that particular signal to be really useful for the same reasons that they might ask me a question on Indirect. It gives me the opportunity to clarify a statement that I have made but believe is misleading or overly broad as it stands.

Trials

Trials are distinctly uncommon because they are expensive, time consuming, stressful and risky for both sides. Settlements are MUCH more common and can occur right up until the day before a trial or, less commonly, during the trial. You are unlikely to be involved in a trial, but most of the points made for deposition apply to the trial as well.

The major differences between a trial and a deposition are:

1. There is a jury. Witnesses generally speak to the jury even though the question comes from a lawyer
2. There is a judge. The judge rules the courtroom. He or she is an absolute potentate during a trial, bound of course by the law. Most judges have earned respect and it is appropriate to address them as "Your Honor."
3. Unlike at the deposition, at trial you do get to "play offense." Your side gets to "tell its story," including all the points you wanted to make at the deposition. If your lawyer calls you as a witness then you tell your story before being questioned by the opposing lawyer. If the opposing lawyer calls you as a witness, then you tell your story afterwards.
4. Although remote testimony is permitted, it is tremendously disadvantageous to your team in terms of interacting with the jury.

Let's reiterate the key points of this chapter for those of you who have continued to the end. First, the best way to learn about the substance of medicolegal actions is to participate in M&M conferences. Second, the best strategy to address medicolegal matters while caring for patients is to ignore them and practice medicine to the best of your ability. Third, if you are involved in a medicolegal action, you should align yourself immediately with your own legal office and be guided by them for all actions and communications. Fourth, if you have to testify, let Aristotelian logic, honesty and simplicity be your guides. Don't answer questions that don't make sense or include unwarranted assumptions or harbor potential traps, and when you do answer, keep it simple and keep it honest.

Chapter 20. Causation in Medicine

This is a fascinating topic that deserves a book of its own. This chapter, however, contains only the briefest possible introduction to the topic. As always, the ideas reflect my own view. The topic is of profound interest to us as clinicians but the first time I really thought seriously about it was when I was serving as an expert defense witness in a class action lawsuit related to testosterone. This was not the first or last time that participation in a legal matter helped improve my thinking and approach to clinical patient care.

I like to start with a capricious scenario and related question.

I am riding my bicycle on a dirt country road on a beautiful Spring day, enjoying nature and happy as a lark. Suddenly, I notice a squirrel running down a tree trunk at the roadside and I swerve in an effort to avoid the squirrel's anticipated next move. As I swerve I hit a rut and go crashing down. (The squirrel never does come into the road.)

The question is, What caused me to fall?

The answer is obvious, but very few give this response.

The answer is that gravity caused me to fall. Without gravity, I wouldn't have fallen.

Hmmm. That seems a bit of a dodge. Not really though.

The point of this story is that causation actually involves two types of factors, not one. First there is one or more predisposing factors which enable an event to occur, making it possible, or even probable, sometime in the future. It "sets the stage" as it were. The second factor is the trigger that actuates the event at a particular moment. Usually, both factors are present when an event occurs.

What caused the patient's intracerebral hemorrhage (ICH)? The patient's PMH includes hypertension for over twenty years. OK, by why did the ICH occur TODAY? Unfortunately, he ran out of his prescription drugs at the beginning of a three day weekend and was unable to get his meds renewed. His BP rose precipitously the day of his ICH. Predisposing Factor: Long-standing sub-optimally controlled hypertension. Trigger: Sudden rise in BP due cessation of medication.

Sometimes either the pre-disposing factor or the trigger is unknown in a given case, it may be a hidden factor or beyond our current scientific understanding. But I have found it very helpful to think about causation for patients by exploring these two factors. A thorough history may already have revealed both the predisposing factor and the trigger. Sometimes, though, upon reflection you cannot identify one or either. That should stimulate you to seek more history and think further. For example, this is the most common way that I diagnose sleep apnea. In a patient with stroke or TIA and physical signs of hypertension but no historical stroke risk factors, the possible answer dawns on me and a few more questions identify the hidden predisposing factor of sleep apnea which worsened recently due to additional weight gain.

Bradford Hill´s Criteria for Relating Causation and Association

The only other topic that I want to introduce in this chapter is Bradford Hill's Criteria for causality. "Hill's Criteria" have evolved over time but the purpose has always been the same and that is to provide explicit guidelines for when a statistical association can be considered as a cause of an event or disease state. I simply want to make you aware of these useful criteria. The following are based on the version from Wikipedia.

Strength (effect size):

The larger the association, the more likely that it is causal. However, a small association does not mean that there is not a causal effect and a large one does not mean that there is.

Consistency (reproducibility):
Consistent findings, observed by different persons in different places and times with different samples, strengthens the likelihood of a causal effect.

Specificity:
Causation is likely if there is a specific population and disease with no other likely explanation. The more specific an association between a factor and an effect is, the greater the probability of a causal relationship.

Temporality:
The effect has to occur after the cause. If there is an expected delay between the cause and expected effect (eg - asbestos exposure), then the effect must occur after that delay.

Biological gradient (dose–response relationship):
Greater exposure should generally lead to greater incidence of the effect. However, in some cases, the mere presence of the factor can trigger the effect.

Plausibility:
A plausible mechanism between cause and effect is helpful but may not be apparent due to limitations of current scientific knowledge.

Coherence:
Coherence between epidemiological and laboratory findings increases the likelihood of an effect. However, lack of laboratory evidence does not nullify the epidemiological associations.

Experiment:
Experimental evidence, like coherence, can increase the likelihood of an effect.

Analogy:
If a similar exposure has been proven to cause a similar outcome in another context, it strengthens the case for a causal link in the current situation, but alone does not establish causation. For example, if there's strong evidence that a particular chemical is teratogenic, then observing a similar dose-response relationship between exposure to a different chemical with a similar structure, could be considered analogous, supporting a potential causal link.

Whether conducting your own research or evaluating the strength of the literature regarding causation of a statistical association with a disease state, the Hill Criteria are valuable guidelines.

A Cautionary Tale
Years ago it was recognized that elevated plasma levels of homocyst(e)ine [H(e)] are strongly associated with endothelial dysfunction and a marked increase in vascular risk. It was also know that treatment with a combination of folic acid, pyridoxine (vitamin B6) and cobalamin (vitamin B12) reduced plasma H(e) levels and improved experimental endothelial function. However, despite high plausibility, there was no direct evidence that such treatment reduced clinical events. The Vitamin Intervention for Stroke Prevention (VISP) trial was conducted to test the hypothesis that reducing H(e) levels would reduce the incidence of stroke and other vascular events in humans. The trial re-demonstrated the associated risk of stroke with higher H(e) and re-demonstrated that H(e) levels could be reduced with the three vitamins, but failed to demonstrate any reduction in stroke or cardiac risk after 4 years. Another factor must be involved and the higher H(e) is more appropriately thought of as a marker of the elevated risk but not causative.

The Hill Criteria strongly favored stroke causation for the elevated H(e) levels, but the VISP trial demonstrated that the H(e) levels *per se* were not the cause of the elevated risk. Direct testing of a hypothesis, when feasible, provides the ultimate criteria for causation.

Chapter 21. Psychiatric Patients

Introduction

This chapter has a single central message along with brief comments on some specific psychiatric disorders.

The central message is: Follow the same principles for your psychiatric patients that you use for all of your other patients. Because their symptoms are behavioral or "mental," many healthcare providers tend to partition psychiatric patients into a separate category. That would imply a mind-body duality which has been rejected since the 17th century. Mental functions are driven by physical forces as much as any other physiologic activity.

There are studies that suggest that, depending on how you define "psychiatric" symptoms, as many as half of all of our patients have psychiatric symptoms or disorders. Most of us have found that the best results occur when you care for patients with psychiatric symptoms using the same principles as for all other patients. Some might argue that the behavioral nature of their symptoms is, somehow, different than other symptoms, but I would simply argue that gastrointestinal symptoms are as different from respiratory symptoms as they are from behavioral symptoms.

There are also several specific points that I would like to share that are based on the wisdom of my teachers and colleagues as well as my own experience with psychiatric patients. I mean why not? Don't Psychiatry and Neurology share a common Board? You may think of the following comments as "psychiatric first aid" while waiting for the help of a psychiatrist. Sometimes first aid is all that the patient needs.

Suggesting a Psychiatric Consult to a Patient

Most patients accept or even welcome the suggestion that we obtain a psychiatric consult but there remains a significant minority who reject the suggestion due to personal or cultural beliefs. For all patients, it makes sense to explain to your patient why you want to involve a psychiatrist, just as you should when you involve any other consultant. My daughter-in-law, Dr. Heather Newman, is a psychiatrist and she recommends including in your reasons to the patient how a psychiatrist can help relieve some of the patient's symptoms such as sleep or appetite disturbance as well as anxiety and depression.

Unfortunately, many patients and families share the misconception that psychiatry is somehow different than other medical conditions and may be resistant to a psychiatric referral. When I encounter such resistance in a patient who I think would benefit from psychiatric evaluation and management, I usually turn the situation around to reflect on me rather than them. "It would be helpful to me if we could involve one of my colleagues from psychiatry. These symptoms must be very stressful. You can't feel good about this, no one would. It's not uncommon for me to ask the help of a psychiatrist and I think it would be really useful. They are simply another kind of doctor, they went to medical school too but they have special training in mental health." Heather would suggest things like "Clearly you are suffering from this . . ." or "You are probably sleep deprived, Psych will help you get better sleep along with helping your other symptoms." Then I'll ask, "So, would it be OK with you if I ask Dr. Smith from Psychiatry to come see you?" This won't guarantee a "Yes" and sometimes it is appropriate for the patient to decline for a variety of reasons. But this approach will decrease the resistance to psychiatry if needed and increase the number of times you hear "OK, that'd be fine" or even "Yes, that would be good." Heather would also say that psychiatry consults are frequently underutilized.

Psychosis

Psychosis simultaneously elicits great sympathy and great fascination, almost curiosity. Encountering a patient with mild psychosis generates a feeling of giddiness, a sense that "something's not right." Being with a patient who has florid psychosis can be uncomfortable and, in exceptional circumstances, carries risk of injury for both the patient and caregivers.

I was taught as a first year medical student that patients with psychosis experience a disturbing sense of loss of control. Mental imagery intrudes into their consciousness in a manner that they cannot control. In one of the most important learning experiences of my training, a psychiatrist taught me that it was possible to reach out mentally to psychotic patients and "offer them a life line." In my teacher's words, "It is as if you say to the patient, without words, that you understand that things are out of control in their world but, in your world, things are very much under control. And you are ready to help steady them in their world by holding their hand and guiding them to a safe place." Wow! Was that really possible? I have learned through many interactions with psychotic patients that it absolutely is possible. In most cases, that "mental hand holding" has enabled the patient to calm down, attend to my words along with those of other providers, and accept parenteral medication such as Haldol to safely end their acute psychosis and permit initiation of oral anti-psychotics. It requires that you consciously relax yourself and offer calm support while remaining alert to your patient's safety as well as your own. Consciously calming yourself is a much better approach than being frazzled, which the patient will surely recognize and which increases their own sense of lack of control.

Heather would also suggest that when the patient is less severely psychotic, or if the patient is experiencing delusions, then there is no point in trying to reason or argue them out of their belief. Rather than exploring "why they believe they have 800 illegitimate children," it would be better to redirect the patient toward exploration of treatable symptoms such as sleep, eating and hygiene.

Depression

Depression is extremely common. Up to 20% of all people experience a major depression during their lifetime. Depression may be obvious or it may be very subtle. Because it is so common and may be so subtle, I have found that the best approach is to routinely ask myself if this patient could be depressed. It is generally safe to dismiss that possibility in a patient who is animated, smiling, interacting enthusiastically and acting purposefully with full cooperation. But lacking those behaviors, I take a moment and reflect on whether the patient's lack of these features is just their personality, or is appropriate to the situation, or is related to subtly altered consciousness. If none of the alternatives fit well, then you need to be alert to the possibility of depression.

Patients with depression usually emote low energy, are poorly animated, express negative thoughts with lack of hope, and give poor effort on exam. It is not uncommon to elicit tears as soon as you "scratch the surface" while exploring the possibility of depression with the patient. But it is often the case that the only sign of depression is a subtle quietness on the part of the patient during your interview and exam. Of course there are many people who are simply quiet and peaceful without depression. Again, being vigilant is the key to recognizing the diagnosis. When you encounter a quiet patient with poor participation, ask yourself if this could reflect depression. I might say to the patient, "You seem very quiet. Is this just how you are or are you feeling down? Are you blue? I wouldn't want to ignore it if you are." They'll let you know and the family may express an opinion as well.

One more perceptive guideline for diagnosing depression, specifically as pseudo-dementia, came from an early colleague of mine, Dr. Arnie Sterman, who pointed out that "people with dementia can't, but people with pseudo-dementia won't try." When you hear your patient respond to your mental status questions with "Who cares?" or "What difference does it make?" or simply dismiss you with a wave of their hand and "I don't know", ask yourself whether this may indicate that the patient is depressed.

Borderline Personality Disorder (BPD)

BPD is a chronic condition which often coexists with other psychiatric conditions. It is characterized by instability. Patients with BPD have an unstable self-image and often have intensely unstable relationships. With this they may demonstrate a fear of abandonment, impulsivity, mood instability and severe stress reactions. Although there has been recent progress with behavioral and cognitive treatments, patients with BPD remain among the most challenging that you will encounter. Part of the reason for this is that borderline patients experiencing heightened stress can engage in non-suicidal self injury as well as an increased risk of attempted suicide. They have also learned to use the implicit or explicit threat of such behaviors as a means of manipulating and retaining the attention of their healthcare providers.

Patients with BPD may present with somatic complaints such as pain, fatigue and vague gastrointestinal issues. If this occurs during fear of abandonment or recent separation, the patient may attempt to use their health providers as substitute for the failing relationship. This can result in prolonged office or ED visits that seem to have no clear direction or resolution. Patients with BPD deserve our understanding, however, since 40-70% of them have experienced sexual, physical or mental abuse earlier in their life. In most cases of BPD that you will encounter, the best response is to sympathetically isolate and address the patient's immediate concerns, manage your time spent with the patient to an appropriate duration, and arrange for psychiatric or psychological assessment or follow-up after discussion with the on-call mental health worker.

Delirium

For the last two decades, the word "delirium" has been used as a synonym for a non-specific encephalopathy. When I was a resident, however, the term had a very specific meaning. It meant that the patient was having behavioral disturbances due to an active mis-perceptions of their environment. This was seen most frequently in *delirium tremens* but also in other conditions. I remember watching a patient who thought and acted as if he was driving a stick shift car while in his ICU bed. And we understood that while a patient's hysterical panic when a nurse approached with a sedative in a syringe didn't make sense in reality, it made perfect sense if the patient perceived the nurse as an attacker wielding a large knife.

The central concept of delirium was that the reaction was appropriate for the patient's perception but that the perception was severely distorted. Unfortunately, there is no longer a word to describe this syndrome. Hopefully, this brief story will serve to help you understand that misperceptions can contribute a great deal to a patient's altered behavior. This syndrome is also relatively common among patients with partial complex epilepsy and related post-ictal states. Unfortunately, we no longer have a word to describe it.

Chapter 22. Interpreting the Literature

Evidence Based Medicine (EBM)

In case you haven't heard, we are in the era of Evidence Based Medicine (EBM). This concept has evolved since it was initially introduced. Quite a few early proponents of EBM were heavily focused on randomized clinical trials, advocating mistrust of all other information, including observational trials and teachings from experienced professors. Gradually, however, this gave way to the current, more reasonable, approach that welcomes all information but recognizes the limitations of each, including the limitations of randomized trials. Also, there is much greater emphasis on the role of judgement in modern EBM because each of us must be able to evaluate both the evidence and the individual patient in order to know which evidence is relevant to each patient.

What do we mean by Evidence?

There are many sources of useful evidence, each with its own advantages and disadvantages. We use all of these sources to create our own "internal data base" of information that we apply during patient care.

Your own personal patient care experience is critically important, growing in value as you care for more and more patients. It is immediate to you and highly individualized, taking into account specific facts of the individual patients contributing to that evidence that could never be conveyed in a scientific report. Of course it can be heavily influenced by bias. I once asked my favorite surgeon what he would do in a particularly complicated patient and he responded, "It depends on how my last case went." I think of my experience as my own personal series of observational studies. Some of my observational series are analogous to Case - Control studies and others are analogous to Cohort studies (see below). We have previously discussed how important it is to be consistent in observing and managing patients in order to learn by applying Osler's Rules.

Considering your experience as EBM data closes the loop on that discussion.

We also can learn from the experience of others. When we discuss patient diagnosis and management with our teachers and our peers we benefit from sharing their experience. There is a trade-off, because we lose a lot of the extreme detail that we obtain from our own direct patient care when we hear the experience of others, but we gain from the enormous increase in the number of cases. Depending on the person we're hearing from, there may be extensive cross-correlations with other data, including what they, in turn, have learned from others. To increase the value of the experiences of others, it is useful to ask questions about how many patients they have seen or treated and how long they followed those patients. This is, basically, what goes on in clinical case conferences as well as during bedside rounds. The more you admire the practice of the physician and their honesty in evaluating their own limitations, the more weight you give to their "evidence" in your internal data base.

Textbooks can also serve as sources of evidence. Their advantage is that they are usually (but not always) written by very experienced practitioners and they usually (but not always) represent well-integrated information presented in a logical manner. They are often out of date, however, especially in actively changing fields. This can be an advantage occasionally, when tracing the history of patient management for a specific condition, but may no longer be relevant to modern patient management. Textbooks are particularly useful in mature fields which are changing slowly.

Educational reviews in peer-reviewed and "throw away" journals are usually closely related to a specific topic and are more up-to-date, but also can be very biased in their presentation so caution is needed. They should never be taken as evidence except in so far as they cite primary research studies or detailed case presentations. As you gain experience, your dependence on texts and reviews as evidence will likely become more limited, except for your favorite textbooks.

The Hierarchy of Evidence in the Literature
At one extreme is descriptive observational evidence. This consists of case reports, small uncontrolled case series and "ecological studies" generated from large databases such as insurance or Federal reports. These are all considered "hypothesis generating." They are useful for suggesting possibilities but do not provide information useful for testing hypotheses or establishing causation. The value of descriptive observational evidence should not be underestimated. For example, the role of MPTP as a cause of Parkinson's disease in the young was first suggested based on descriptive observational studies and then developed through basic research using animal, *in vitro* and biochemical models. Obviously, it would not be ethical to conduct a randomized, blinded clinical trial (RCT).

At the other hierarchical extreme are the RCTs and meta-analyses restricted to RCTs which provide the strongest evidence available for testing hypotheses. The complexity of establishing causation has already been discussed through Hill's Criteria and the VISP trial. RCTs are the gold standard for establishing associations which lay the foundation for patient management and establishing causation. There is a recent wonderful move toward "pragmatic" RCTs that permit more flexible and efficient trial designs. These meet the criteria for RCTs but also solve many of the problems of conventional RCTs. Meta-analyses may enhance the value of randomized, controlled blinded studies when the previously published primary studies are relatively homogeneous so that apples can be compared to apples and the number of subjects is increased. But care is needed in evaluating them because the data becomes weaker if the studies are heterogeneous or if observational studies are included. There are published criteria for evaluating meta-analyses. Even greater caution is needed when interpreting "systematic reviews" since that term implies that the publication did not meet the criteria of a meta-analysis. Don't get me wrong, systematic reviews can be very useful but they are not an RCT and they are not a meta-analysis. I think of them as mainly educational.

"In between" is, as usual, in between. The level of evidence includes analytical observational studies. Analytical observational studies include Case-Control and Cohort designs that are considered to provide support for a hypothesis. Depending on the design and data (consistency of data collection, sample size, sample homogeneity, selection criteria, length of follow-up), the support may be weak or strong. So why do we use these types of design? To begin with, it is not always possible to conduct an RCT. The evidence that cigarette smoking causes cancer and COPD is a good example, the story of MPTP is another. You cannot design an ethical RCT. Surgical procedures can be tough as well. How far do you go with the sham procedure? Do you operate and expose the problem that prompted the surgery but not try to correct it? Clearly, there are ethical limits here that can make blinding very difficult. Sometimes an RCT is feasible ethically but unreasonably expensive for its benefit to society, perhaps the necessary sample size is too large, etc. Furthermore, RCT's can take so long to complete (5 years or more would not be unusual) that the field has already moved on to newer diagnostic or treatment techniques. The good news is that well conducted observational studies can provide evidence that is nearly as good as randomized trials although never fully equivalent because it is impossible to absolutely eliminate bias. They can be very valuable supporting the results of a single or smaller RCT. Sometimes they are the strongest evidence obtainable under the circumstances.

Both analytical observational study designs are intended to establish whether there is an association between an "exposure" and an "event" in a particular group of patients, such as those with a specific disease. The exposure may be a drug, a procedure, an environmental exposure or a disease. The event is a definable outcome such as a drug complication, survival to some fixed time point or a measure of quality of life. The essential difference between Case-Control and Cohort studies centers around the 'direction of enquiry.'

In Case-Control studies, patients are recruited because the patient has experienced the outcome (Case) or has not experienced the outcome

(Control). Ideally, except for having experienced the outcome, Cases and Controls should be closely matched. The direction of enquiry then moves backwards in time from outcome to exposure. In both groups, medical records are reviewed to establish whether the patient did or did not meet the criteria for exposure. After appropriate data tabulation and analysis, the study then compares the frequency of exposure amongst the Cases and Controls and compares the probability that Cases (patients with the outcome) and Controls met exposure criteria. The results are typically reported as the Odds ratio of exposure between the two groups. Note that patients are selected because they experienced an outcome (and matched to those who did not) and then the prior medical records are reviewed to establish whether there was an exposure to the factor of interest in both groups. The net result is, fundamentally, a 2X2 table.

Case-Control studies are efficient for the study of rare diseases, requiring smaller sample sizes. They can evaluate multiple risk factors in one study and may be the only feasible study design for very rare diseases. However, they are inefficient for rare exposures, the timing of exposure and outcome may not be clear, and they are subject to selection and recall bias.

In Cohort studies, subjects are identified on the basis of the presence or absence of the exposure of interest. The direction of enquiry then moves forward in time.

Cohort studies can be conducted prospectively or retrospectively. When prospective, the patient is identified and followed clinically, with enrollment in the study either right before or after exposure but prior to the outcome of interest. When retrospective, patients with the exposure of interest are identified within a medical record system and then the initial and subsequent charted visits are reviewed to identify when there was exposure as well as if and when the outcome event occurred. In Cohort studies, the temporal relationship between exposure and disease is clear and permits ascertainment of incidence, not just prevalence (which is not true in the Case-Control study).

Obviously a prospective clinical study is not possible with the Case-Control design.

Cohort studies are particularly good for studying rare exposures and allow maximal investigator control over case finding, exposure classification and follow-up. When prospective and done well, they may approximate RCT for reliable data and reliable evidence. However, they are large, time consuming and expensive when prospective. Retrospective studies are weaker and only slightly better than hypothesis generating. The long time means that exposure may evolve over time and loss to follow-up can be problematic.

An Example

In order to compare the various types of evidence more fully, let's explore an example used by the AAN committee which designed an EBM course for Neurology residents.

Case Report

You are treating a patient who has Parkinson's disease with a dopamine agonist and notice that he has developed valvular heart disease since you met him. Strange, right? So you write a case report about this one patient and suggest the hypothesis that dopamine agonists may lead to valvular heart disease. No proof here, could be a coincidence, just an idea.

Case Series

You spotted another case report of a Parkinson's patient who developed cardiac valvular disease while on dopamine agonist therapy. You have access to medical records for a large population of patient's with Parkinson's disease and decide to search the case files. You find a dozen patients who were found to have cardiac valvular disease while taking dopamine agonists. You publish a case series. This is certainly stronger than a case report but hardly proof of an association given the small number, incomplete and non-standardized data collection and potential for referral bias.

Ecological Association

Several epidemiologists notice your case series and crunch data for a European Union data base. They notice that in countries where sales of dopamine agonists are high, the rate of valvular heart disease in Parkinson's patients is high. Clearly this adds a population ("ecological") basis to suggest an association, but the database contains no link between use and illness nor any information about timing. This also cannot provide proof but strengthens the case to conduct further studies to test for an association.

Case-Control Study

A team of investigators have noticed these case reports and ecological data and decide to work together to identify a group of Parkinson's disease patients who also have cardiac valvular disease (the Cases). They identify an analogous group of Parkinson's disease patients who do not have evidence of a cardiac valvulopathy at the same institutions (the Controls). The frequency of exposure to dopamine agonist therapy is then determined by review of medical and pharmacy records for all subjects.

In this published Case-Control study, it was found that dopamine agonist exposure occured more frequently in Parkinson's disease patients who have cardiac valvulopathy than amongst those who do not. Patients with Parkinson's disease and valvular heart disease had an odds 8.78 times higher of having been treated with a dopamine agonist than patients with Parkinson's disease who did not have valvular heart disease. Those are very steep odds for this association to be by chance alone and the movement disorder community takes notice.

Cohort Study

In order to undertake a prospective Cohort study, investigators would identify a population of patients with Parkinson's disease, some of whom have been exposed to dopamine agonists and some not. All subjects should be free of the outcome (i.e. not have any evidence for cardiac valve disease) at the time of entry into the study;

the patients would then be followed in clinic forward in time to identify those who go on to develop cardiac valvulopathy. As obvious potential sources of bias for this study, however, you can imagine that some local physicians may stop their patients′dopamine agonists after reading the Case-Control report and others might refer any patient who develops a valvulopathy to the clinic because they know of the investigators' interest. Furthermore, it wouldn't be possible to exclude a treatment bias in which certain patients had an unrecognized feature which stimulated their physicians to use dopamine agonists. None of these potential sources of bias can be excluded without an RCT.

Any chance of doing a Cohort study or even an RCT? Given the odds found on the Case-Control study, the cost, and the risk of continuing to use dopamine agonists while awaiting the results, I would say not. And we are hardly at equipoise. I also think it is worth commenting that one exciting use of Bayesian statistics is that you could calculate how much additional negative information would be needed to overcome the suspicion of harm that already exists based on the Case-Control study. It is a sophisticated calculation but readily within the capability of modern statisticians using modern statistical software.

Anyway, this example has always struck me as particularly helpful for understanding observational studies and the nature of evidence. I hope it helps you.

Some Practical Thoughts on How We Use Evidence

I search the literature about 15 times on a normal day. Even after 44 years in practice? Absolutely! There are many reasons go to the literature.

A. Things I don't know

There are many times that I want particular information to help with decision making and I don't have the answer; there are times that I hear others mention something that I have never heard of or have heard of only in passing.

B. Things I think I know but want to be sure

Often, I have known about a field, have used concepts and specifics in the field, but a pending decision depends critically on the accuracy of my memory. That's not good enough for patient care. I want to confirm what I think I know.

C. Things I know but want to make sure I am up to date

There are times that I am quite confident in what I know but I haven't methodically reviewed a field or a specific question in that field in more than a couple of years. I want to find out if there have been any new developments, especially new forms of treatment, that I may have missed in my regular reading.

D. Things I want to share with others

There are many times when I am confident in my knowledge and very up to date but I want to make others aware of what I know pertinent to a patient we are sharing. It may be that there is an opportunity to teach or there may be a difference in opinion related to the patient's care. In that case, I go to the literature to find an article which illustrates the points that I want to make. That may involve a well-written primary research article or a current review.

So get used to it. You will be using the literature heavily throughout your career. It is an important skill to use proficiently and efficiently. The need for information may occur in the middle of the day when things are already very hectic, so efficiency is very important. No doubt AI will improve our searches in the near future (or is already doing so) but I think it will be a while before you can rely entirely on AI to provide exactly the information you want, including a sense ofd the strength of the evidence, without having it unintentionally introduce bias. And you will still have to exert judgement to decide if the information applies to your patient.

How Do I "Read" an Article?

My literature searching supplements my regular reading. I remain current in my field by reading 6 journals regularly. My general medical knowledge is supported by reading the New England Journal of Medicine and the Medical Letter. I recommend both for every practicing internist, including neurologists. To remain current in neurology, pediatric neurology and translational advances in neuroscience, I read Neurology and the Annals of Neurology. For my sub-specialties, I read Stroke and Neurocritical Care.

How is it possible to keep up with this many journals in addition to 15 searches a day for as-needed information while engaging in a busy practice?

Here is how I approach an article. First, I use speed reading skills. Rather than plod one word at a time, it is faster and more effective to skim read quickly and then pause to ask yourself what you just read. If something isn't clear, search for related words in what you just skimmed and give that more attention. Secondly, the fundamental question is how far to keep reading an article. How much time do I allocate to any article? In a sense, I am always looking for reasons to stop reading this article and move onto the next. The three most common reasons to stop are that A) the article is not relevant to my practice, B) it was great and I already have my answer from it, and C) it's a good article but there is nothing in it that is new to me (this reason definitely increases over time).

In most cases, I consciously read in a consistent pattern although the pattern can vary flexibly. Also, routine reading and as-needed reading from a search can differ although there are basic similarities. First the title. Is this paper likely to address my needs? No? Stop! Yes or Maybe, onto the Conclusion in the Abstract. Is it worth exploring the basis for this conclusion? If the conclusion isn't explicit, then up to Abstract Results. Same question. Worth the time to know the basis of the primary result? If it is, then onto a detailed read of the Abstract's Methods and Results. Then ask yourself, do you really need to know more about this subject? If not, move on. Sometimes, however, the answer is a resounding Yes. In that case, begin reading the text of the article, slowing down or speeding up, depending on how relevant the particular information is to your practice or to your specific question. Need more information, use the References to explore the topic further. Sometimes, the only thing I want from an article in my routine reading is a mechanism of action of a "novel therapeutic agent" along with the trial design and results. This typically applies in a field that is somewhat remote from my practice but one that became an interest for some particular reason. I like to remain current on the newest therapeutic and diagnostic principles even though I may not use them. You never know when they might come in handy. In that case, I read the Abstract Introduction, or the paper's Introduction or the paper's Discussion until I find the drug's mechanism of action or the basis of the novel procedure. I might barely skim the rest of the paper except to see in Results how much better the new approach is compared to the one that I already knew, presumably the trial's active control.

When reviewing a whole collection of articles which appear in an as-needed literature search, it is especially necessary to move efficiently. So keep asking, A) Does it address my question? B) How and how well does it address my question? C) Do I have enough evidence from this and the others or do I need to keep reading more articles?

When you are reading an article that is very relevant to your field or for an as-needed question, there are additional pieces of necessary information. For example, I am considering using a new treatment or diagnostic measure in my practice. This is an important matter so I need some very specific information. First, to what population does this paper apply exactly? Is the information relevant to my patient or patients? Secondly, how effective is the treatment or the test relative to my prior approaches? Third, what are the safety concerns? Fourth, is it feasible within my available resources, that is, in my medical center? Fifth, is there anyone that I know who would be accessible in person or by phone who might already have experience with this modality "whose brain I can pick?"

PICO

A valuable and simple tool to help initiate a literature search uses the mnemonic aid PICO which stands for Patient - Intervention - Comparator - Outcome.

You can make the patient category as general or specific as you like, as general as {stroke} or as specific as {stroke AND acute AND ischemic AND female AND pregnant}. The intervention might be a single therapy such as TNK or broader such as {TNK OR TPA OR thrombolysis OR mechanical thrombectomy OR bridging therapy}. The comparator also could be a single agent {aspirin} or multiple {aspirin OR anti-platelet OR anti-coagulation OR heparin OR NOAC OR warfarin}. The outcome can be general {human} or specific {(infant OR newborn) AND (mortality OR bleeding complications OR Rankin score OR survival OR IQ OR quality of life)}.

You build this in a standard PUBMED format using the Advanced option, creating the four PICO components separately and then assembling them as the final search. You can even specify which section of the article should contain your search terms.

For example, to investigate the safety of TNK for fetuses of pregnant women treated for acute stroke you might use the following search in PICO format.

Patient: {STROKE AND ACUTE AND ISCHEMIC AND PREGNANT}
AND
Intervention: {TNK}
AND
Comparison: {ASPIRIN OR ANTIPLATELET OR HEPARIN}
AND
Outcome: {ABORTION OR MISCARRIAGE OR INFANT MORTALITY OR NEONATAL ICU OR TERATOGENICITY OR PERIVENTRICULAR HEMORRHAGE}.

When searching for diagnostic modalities, the Patient is unchanged. The intervention is the imaging modality of interest and the comparator is the second (or second, third and fourth) modalities. The outcome would typically be {Sensitivity OR Specificity}.

To investigate the use of MRI for coronary ischemia with the PICO format the search might look something like this.

Patient: {ANGINA OR CORONARY ISCHEMIA OR MI OR MYOCARDIAL INFARCTION OR CAD OR CORONARY ARTERY DISEASE}
AND
Intervention: {MRI}
AND
Comparison: {CORONARY ANGIOGRAPHY OR CARDIAC CATHETERIZATION OR PCI}
AND
Outcome: {SENSITIVITY OR SPECIFICITY OR ACCURACY}.

Extracting Information from a Research Paper

Let's assume that you have found several articles pertinent to your question of interest and that after your initial review you have chosen a few peer reviewed articles that you want to use to answer your question because they are pertinent to your patients and the techniques are feasible for your practice. You have already read these articles from start to finish. How do you evaluate the information and extract what is useful to you?

Remember that we evaluate evidence for inductive reasoning not as valid or invalid but as relatively stronger or weaker. What factors contribute to stronger evidence?

A primary determinant of strength of evidence is based on the study design of the paper. As already discussed, in increasing order of strength, there are descriptive observational studies, analytic observational studies and prospective, randomized trials and meta-analyses. For all of these, it is essential that the research questions or objectives are clearly defined and that the design is appropriate for the objectives. Details of experimental design are important and formal evaluation criteria are available for evaluating designs.

Within any of these categories, in general, studies with more patients and followed for a longer period of time provide stronger evidence. Of course, the metrics that are used have to be appropriate for the question being addressed.

While conducting a study and writing a paper are two very different skills, it is usually the case that a well-written paper predicts a carefully executed study. Ideally, the paper lays out the justification, methods and results of the research in a clear and logical manner. A question that I like to ask myself is whether I could reproduce the study or experiment based on the information provided. If I have unanswered questions about how to repeat the study, then I must have some uncertainty about the methods that were used and therefore about the reliability of the results as well.

Key information for any clinical study should be available in "Figure 1," including the number of screened subjects who were enrolled and the number of subjects lost to follow-up. It is generally considered that a study which has lost follow-up for 20% or more of the enrolled subjects is not reliable. The VISP study lost only 1% of its subjects to follow-up, some sites did not lose any. Even 10% of subjects lost to follow-up raises important questions in my mind about the oversight and overall conduct of the study. Even if the reasons for loss of follow-up are specified and understandable, it is still the case that the loss of subjects introduces greater risk of bias.

Most published trials provide a detailed review, in Figure 1, demonstrating the entire process of subject participation with numbers and explanations. This includes everything from screening, reasons for failure to enroll, adherence to randomization, cross-overs, subjects lost to follow-up and subjects who completed the study. Outcomes are not included. This figure is the easiest way to learn about the overall conduct of the study and provides useful insight into the strength of the investigation.

Other useful questions for evaluating the value of the research for your practice are whether the objectives have been answered, whether the authors have limited their conclusions based on their patient population and the effect size, outcome measures and results and whether there are any potential confounding influences that may explain the results and that are not related to the research question. A quick check of author conflicts of interest is usually a good idea to gauge the potential for favoritism bias, especially if there are potential financial implications from the results in terms of the sale of drugs or procedural equipment.

It is important to maintain focus on the question of whether the research applies to your patients. You chose to give the article detailed attention because you believed that it did. But did it? A necessary trade off of study design has to do with the generalizability of the research. "Proof of concept" studies generally focus narrowly on a homogeneous population in order to minimize subject variability but this may limit the type of patients to which the current results apply. At the opposite extreme, the results for the study may be obtained from a population so broad that you are not sure whether there were sub-groups very different from your patient that dominated the overall results and conclusions. It may help if sub-group analyses have been included. Sometimes inter-group interactions are reported. It is particularly important to note which patients were excluded. For example, critical carotid stenoses (>90% or >95%) were routinely excluded from early randomized carotid endarterectomy trials because of lack of equipoise and safety concerns. While it was natural for clinicians to extend the trial results to those with higher degrees of stenosis, the scientific justification for doing so were dubious at best and this important group has been addressed primarily with analytical observational studies and practitioner experience.

It is important to appreciate the effect size of the study results. Statistical evaluation of chance is not the same as effect size. It is possible to identify a small effect with a very high degree of statistical certainty but the effect size may be so small that the treatment is not worth the trouble. How important was the outcome? If you knew with high degree of certainty that intensive chemotherapy increased your patient's life expectancy by half a month, would that be worth the side effects and effort required for the chemotherapy? If the study demonstrated with high confidence that monthly headaches were reduced from 15 to 12, would your patient be willing to introduce another twice daily medication or forgo alternative therapies? Clearly the magnitude of benefit based on the chosen outcome measures is important.

It is also important to recognize the difference between relative benefit and absolute benefit. For a rare outcome, a small absolute reduction of that outcome may be associated with a high relative improvement in outcome. For example, if an outcome occurs 7 times in a control sample population of 1000 and the treatment reduces the number of outcomes to 5 in 1000 subjects, the relative risk reduction is (7-5)/7 = 28%, but the absolute risk reduction is (7-5)/1000, or 0.2%. Hmmm.

The most useful values to guide clinical decisions are usually the number needed to treat (NNT) and the associated number needed to harm (NNH). Mechanical thrombectomy within 6 hours of the onset of acute ischemic stroke yields one additional patient who achieves independence for every three patients treated; the NNT, is 3. That's exceptional! For patients with asymptomatic carotid stenosis, it was shown with a high level of confidence that you would have to operate on 127 patients to prevent one stroke, the NNT = 127. That's not so great. Would you recommend mechanical thrombectomy? How about endarterectomy?

It also goes without saying that the NNT must be smaller than the NNH. So, giving IV tPA to patients between 4.5 and 6 hours after onset of acute ischemic stroke has an NNT of about 16 but the NNH is closer to 10. Would you use tPA at 6 hours after stroke onset based on that data? Obviously, not since you are more likely to do harm than good, assuming roughly equal value to the benefit and harm.

This issue of relative value of complications is more relevant than you might think. In trials of carotid endarterectomy vs carotid stenting, both the NNT to prevent stroke and the NNH are essentially the same in the two treatment groups but the complications in the endarterectomy group are primarily myocardial infarction, often asymptomatic and diagnosed by blood tests, while the complications of the stenting group are stroke and death. Details matter. Fortunately, the NNH is very high in both groups (complications are not common) but the distinction is worth noting and is relevant to patient and procedure selection.

I would like to end this chapter where we started. While, reading the literature involves a lot of technical knowledge and practice, the most important aspect is not based on statistics, methods or experimental design. The most important question is whether this paper applies to your patients and to your practice. This involves judgement on your part. There is no substitute for it. So from the point that you start reading until you finish reading, you should continuously be asking yourself "Does this apply to my patients?" If not, take away what is interesting and move on. There is always plenty of work to do and plenty of people waiting to have fun with you.

Epilogue

Congratulations, you have reached the end of the book! I hope you enjoyed it and found it useful.

I would be glad to hear from you. Feel free to send any comments or suggestions, or any stories you want to share, directly to me, at newmang.einstein@gmail.com.

I hope that you have a long and successful career. I mean that I hope you retire many years from now as a happy, experienced physician, loved by your patients, colleagues and students; missed in your community; happy that you chose medicine as a career; and leaving the field satisfied that you have helped many, many patients.

www.ingramcontent.com/pod-product-compliance
Lightning Source LLC
LaVergne TN
LVHW052036200926
848481LV00005B/1698

* 9 7 9 8 9 9 3 5 5 3 2 0 7 *